Empathy in the Treatment of Trauma and PTSD

BRUNNER-ROUTLEDGE PSYCHOSOCIAL STRESS SERIES
Charles R. Figley, Ph.D., Series Editor

1. Stress Disorders among Vietnam Veterans, Edited by Charles R. Figley, Ph.D.
2. Stress and the Family Vol. 1: Coping with Normative Transitions, Edited by Hamilton I. McCubbin, Ph.D. and Charles R. Figley, Ph.D.
3. Stress and the Family Vol. 2: Coping with Catastrophe, Edited by Charles R. Figley, Ph.D., and Hamilton I. McCubbin, Ph.D.
4. Trauma and Its Wake: The Study and Treatment of Post-Traumatic Stress Disorder, Edited by Charles R. Figley, Ph.D.
5. Post-Traumatic Stress Disorder and the War Veteran Patient, Edited by William E. Kelly, M.D.
6. The Crime Victim's Book, Second Edition, By Morton Bard, Ph.D., and Dawn Sangrey.
7. Stress and Coping in Time of War: Generalizations from the Israeli Experience, Edited by Norman A. Milgram, Ph.D.
8. Trauma and Its Wake Vol. 2: Traumatic Stress Theory, Research, and Intervention, Edited by Charles R. Figley, Ph.D.
9. Stress and Addiction, Edited by Edward Gottheil, M.D., Ph.D., Keith A. Druley, Ph.D., Steven Pashko, Ph.D., and Stephen P. Weinsteinn, Ph.D.
10. Vietnam: A Casebook, by Jacob D. Lindy, M.D., in collaboration with Bonnie L. Green, Ph.D., Mary C. Grace, M.Ed., M.S., John A. MacLeod, M.D., and Louis Spitz, M.D.
11. Post-Traumatic Therapy and Victims of Violence, Edited by Frank M. Ochberg, M.D.
12. Mental Health Response to Mass Emergencies: Theory and Practice, Edited by Mary Lystad, Ph.D.
13. Treating Stress in Families, Edited by Charles R. Figley, Ph.D.
14. Trauma, Transformation, and Healing: An Integrative Approach to Theory, Research, and Post-Traumatic Therapy, By John P. Wilson, Ph.D.
15. Systemic Treatment of Incest: A Therapeutic Handbook, By Terry Trepper, Ph.D., and Mary Jo Barrett, M.S.W.
16. The Crisis of Competence: Transitional Stress and the Displaced Worker, Edited by Carl A. Maida, Ph.D., Norma S. Gordon, M.A., and Norman L. Farberow, Ph.D.
17. Stress Management: An Integrated Approach to Therapy, by Dorothy H. G. Cotton, Ph.D.
18. Trauma and the Vietnam War Generation: Report of the Findings from the National Vietnam Veterans Readjustment Study, By Richard A. Kulka, Ph.D., William E. Schlenger, Ph.D., John A. Fairbank, Ph.D., Richard L. Hough, Ph.D., Kathleen Jordan, Ph.D., Charles R. Marmar, M.D., Daniel S. Weiss, Ph.D., and David A. Grady, Psy.D.
19. Strangers at Home: Vietnam Veterans Since the War, Edited by Charles R. Figley, Ph.D., and Seymour Leventman, Ph.D.
20. The National Vietnam Veterans Readjustment Study: Tables of Findings and Technical Appendices, By Richard A. Kulka, Ph.D., Kathleen Jordan, Ph.D., Charles R. Marmar, M.D., and Daniel S. Weiss, Ph.D.
21. Psychological Trauma and the Adult Survivor: Theory, Therapy, and Transformation, By I. Lisa McCann, Ph.D., and Laurie Anne Pearlman, Ph.D.
22. Coping with Infant or Fetal Loss: The Couple's Healing Process, By Kathleen R. Gilbert, Ph.D., and Laura S. Smart, Ph.D.
23. Compassion Fatigue: Coping with Secondary Traumatic Stress Disorder in Those Who Treat the Traumatized, Edited by Charles R. Figley, Ph.D.
24. Treating Compassion Fatigue, Edited by Charles R. Figley, Ph.D.
25. Handbook of Stress, Trauma and the Family, Edited by Don R. Catherall, Ph.D.
26. The Pain of Helping: Psychological Injury of Helping Professionals, by Patrick J. Morrissette, Ph.D., RMFT, NCC, CCC
27. Disaster Mental Health Services: A Primer for Practitioners, by Diane Myers, R.N., M.S.N, and David Wee, M.S.S.W.

Editorial Board

EMPATHY IN THE TREATMENT OF TRAUMA AND PTSD

JOHN P. WILSON, PH.D.
RHIANNON BRWYNN THOMAS, PH.D., B.C.E.T.S.

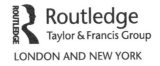

Routledge
Taylor & Francis Group

LONDON AND NEW YORK

First published in 2004 by
Brunner-Routledge
Taylor & Francis Group

Published 2014 by
Routledge
771 Third Avenue,
New York, NY 10017

Published in Great Britain by
Routledge
27 Church Road, Hove,
East Sussex BN3 2FA, UK

First issued in paperback 2014

Routledge is an imprint of the Taylor and Francis Group, an informa business

Library of Congress Cataloging-in-Publication Data

Wilson, John. P. (John Preston)
  Empathy in the treatment of trauma and PTSD/John P. Wilson, Rhiannon B. Thomas.
   p. ; cm. — (Brunner-Routledge psychosocial stress series)
   Includes bibliographical references and index.
   ISBN 978-0-415-94758-9 (hardback : alk. paper)
   1. Psychic trauma—Treatment. 2. Post-traumatic stress disorder—Treatment.
  3. Empathy. 4. Psychotherapist and patient.
    [DNLM: 1. Psychotherapeutic Processes. 2. Empathy. 3. Professional-Patient
  Relations. 4. Stress Disorders, Post-Traumatic—therapy. WM 420 W752e 2004]
  I. Thomas, Rhiannon B. II. Title. III. Series.

RC552.T7W557 2004
616.85'2106—dc22   2004006641

ISBN 978-0-415-94758-9 (hbk)
ISBN 978-1-138-87157-1 (pbk)

Dedication

This book is dedicated to William and Martha Butterfield, whose lives have exemplified the highest forms of empathy with compassionate caring for those whose lives have been touched by them.

Contents

Foreword

Jerome (assumed name) was doing his utmost to understand what the client was saying to him. Everyone in the observation room, his fellow doctoral students enrolled in the trauma practicum and I intently watched the TV screen, which was connected, through closed circuit, to the cameras in the room down the hall.

"You are angry that the police took so long to rescue you," Jerome said with hope in his voice. Hope that this time, after three attempts, Sarah (assumed name) would reply in relief, "Yes!" Instead the young woman stared at him, then looked down, shook her head and said, "Not really. I was mostly angry at myself that I got myself into being assaulted by the jerk, b ..." Jerome jumped in, " ... because you should have known that he would attack you?" Sarah just stared, as if hoping that Jerome was joking or trying to cheer her. It was as obvious to her as it was to us that Jerome had no clue to her real feelings. Jerome was angry at Sarah's former boyfriend for hurting her. He would never have allowed such abuse in his own life and could not understand why she had allowed this to come about. Jerome would "have killed the guy," as he explained in group supervision at the end of the day's sessions. Jerome admitted that he did not "connect" well with Sarah; that he felt lost during the session and desperate to understand what she was saying to him, and he was searching for an approach to help her "solve" her problem.

Training the next generation of therapists for work with the traumatized is both a challenge and a privilege. One of the most important ingredients for a successful trainee and therapist is establishing a solid therapeutic alliance with the client. To do this requires not only careful listening but also sensing, using one's entire being. "Listening" to the client, in an effort to build such a vital alliance and utilize it in servicing the client, demands an extraordinary facility for empathy. And to achieve this requires the full resources of the therapist's "self." At the same time, it is important to protect the therapist's self from being traumatized in the service of the traumatized. Who better to do this than Drs. John P. Wilson and Rhiannon B. Thomas?

The book is divided into 11 chapters, evolving from a discussion of the unconscious transmission of trauma in chapter 1 to, finally, a chapter that discusses effective empathic attunement in service to the traumatized client. A special bonus is the inclusion of the Clinicians' Trauma Reaction Survey Questionnaire. This allows the reader to evaluate her or his own reactivity tendencies and how they compare with others that Wilson and Thomas have studied over the last decade of research in this area.

This book represents both a paradigm shift toward a new approach to trauma treatment and, at the same time, a celebration of the paradigm adopted by a majority of earlier practitioners in the field. The new paradigm involves immersion into the client's "phenomenal reality and ego-space" in order to reach "empathic attunement." This attunement is the "capacity to resonate efficiently and accurately to another's state of being," which means understanding the client's world, including the client's world schema and internal psychological ego states. Wilson and Thomas boldly assert that empathic ability, including empathic attunement, is a *requirement* for effective post-traumatic or traumatology psychotherapy. Empathic attunement enables the therapist to detect and accurately translate the multiple "signals" or messages from the client.

In language that is almost mystical, Wilson and Thomas draw attention to " … energy in wave form emanating from the trauma client and manifesting themselves in various amplitudes and frequencies as they 'flow' in patterns towards the receptor site of the therapist's mind and consciousness." Using this analogy of communication, the co-authors point out that the therapist must have a capacity for constantly decoding and encoding in a fine-tuned sequence of interactions. This requires that considerable clinical skill be focused on the client's needs and awareness of the therapist's self.

Drawing from Wilson's book written a decade earlier, the co-authors define empathy as "the psychological capacity to identify and understand another person's psychological state of being." Empathic attunement, then, enables the therapist to connect and calibrate with the client's being in the most effective and efficient way possible. Wilson and Thomas also point out that the use of empathy, though vitally important, is only one of several means of connecting to the client's being, both conscious and unconscious (i.e., ego-state and unconscious process). They point to seven separate channels of information exchanged between client and therapist in the context of the session and their emerging therapeutic alliance. They suggest that these channels enable the transmission of information or signals between client and therapist. The channels are affect, defense, somatic state, ego-states, personality, unconscious memory and cognitive processes. The co-authors indicate that information is transmitted from client to therapist, who receives the transmission and then decodes it for use in the treatment process.

Why is this useful? By viewing the transmission of information in this way, Wilson and Thomas can show the importance of empathic attunement as a vehicle for accurate reception of the information being generated by the patient. Thus, the trauma worker's therapeutic effectiveness and proper management of his or her self demands that he or she operate on all channels, accurately receiving and decoding information and possessing the ability and capacity to manage this information for use in the therapeutic process.

Returning to the case example noted in the beginning of this foreword, Jerome was making every effort to understand what Sarah was saying to him. In addition to focusing on appearing competent to his fellow trainee therapists and their supervisor, Jerome was desperate to be a good therapist and to "listen" to his client. Jerome endeavored to be empathic and was at a loss to explain why his efforts were not working out. He later developed the skill and psychological capacity to identify and understand his client's psychological state of being. Through practice, self-reflection and patience, he was able to calibrate his empathic attunement so as to almost connect and calibrate with his client's being — not just relate to what the client was *saying*.

I hope that this book serves as a change agent for all of the psychotherapy training programs like ours at Florida State University, to shift from a paradigm of cookbook, how to, psychotherapy training to a far more integrative and holistic approach represented in this excellent study. By being more attuned to the dynamic, interactional, multiple channels of communication between therapist and client and the critical role of the therapist's self, we improve not only the quality of psychotherapy practice but also the quality of life of those who practice it. Listening to clients who have been traumatized is very challenging work, leaving fingerprints on the heart which are sometimes difficult to manage or erase. This book helps us become aware of the therapeutic process for the mutual benefit of the helper and the helped.

Charles R. Figley, Ph.D.
Series Editor

Acknowledgments

Our appreciation and thanks extend to many people who have helped bring this book to life.

First, the senior author gratefully acknowledges the support of the J. William Fulbright Foundation and the opportunity to serve as a Fulbright Scholar at the University of Zagreb Medical School in 2003–2004. Dr. Rudolf Gregurek of the medical school faculty was an especially supportive Fulbright sponsor who encouraged work on the ideas developed for the book.

Our special thanks to Professor Joel Aronoff of Michigan State University who provided encouragement and incisive critiques of early drafts of the book; and to Charles R. Figley of Florida State University and editor of the Brunner-Routledge Psychosocial Stress Series for his support of the project.

We express appreciation of the encouragement we received from Emily Epstein-Loeb, associate editor at Brunner-Routledge, who was instrumental in overseeing the inception and production of the book itself.

We also gratefully acknowledge the tireless dedication of Kathleen D. Letizio, whose willingness to oversee the production of the book's many versions brought this work to fruition. Kathy made sure that the book was word processed to perfection. She labored at a distance, periodically receiving Federal Express boxes of the original manuscript from Zagreb, Croatia and rapidly transforming them into chapters which were then returned by e-mail on dozens of occasions until the final version was in place. Her professional dedication and understanding of post-traumatic stress disorder reflect her empathy and compassion as a person.

Finally, we acknowledge the support of Cleveland State University and Dr. Mark Ashcraft of the Department of Psychology; and we thank the International Society of Dissociative Disorders and the International Society for Traumatic Stress Studies for assisting in the research study reported in chapters 7 and 9.

1

The Transmitting Unconscious of Traumatization

Listen to the voices of trauma. Can you hear their cry? Their pain exudes emotional blood from psychic pores. Nights are broken by frightening intrusions from ghosts of the past. Bodies hold memories, secrets and scars locked into sinew, glands and neurons. Weary souls of the abyss seeking peace in their souls.

John P. Wilson, 2003

INTRODUCTION

Trauma is part of the human condition and ever present in the lives of ordinary people throughout the world. Traumatic events punctuate recorded history in a manner parallel to momentous achievements which advance civilization. Such events are the product of human intentions, the randomness of nature and acts of God.

Trauma is archetypal in nature and has its own psychological structure and energy (Wilson, 2002, 2003). Traumatic experiences vary along many different *stressor* dimensions and have simple and complex effects on the human psyche (Wilson, 2004; Wilson & Lindy, 1994). Such episodes are not only different qualitatively and quantitatively from one another, but they are also subjectively experienced in individual ways through the life history of the victim, the filters of culture and language, and the nature of injury afflicting the organism in all of its integrated wholeness. Trauma may strike at the surface or the deepest core of the self — the very soul and innermost identity of the person. Traumatic ordeals may lead to transformations of the personality, spirit, beliefs, and understanding of the meaning of life. In that same sense, these experiences alter life-course trajectories and have multigenerational legacies (Danieli, 1988). In a broader perspective, massive or catastrophic trauma may permanently change, damage or eradicate entire societies, cultures and nations (Lifton, 1967, 1993). As an archetypal form, trauma can be a psychic force of enormous power in the individual and collective unconscious of the

1

species. Unmetabolized trauma of a violent nature caused by wars, terrorism, torture, genocide, ethnic cleansing, and the purposeful abuse of others may unleash destructive forces within the fabric of civilization (Freud, 1917, 1928; Jung, 1929; Wilson, Friedman & Lindy, 2001).

Trauma that is unhealed, unresolved and unintegrated into a healthy balance within the self has the potential to be repeated, reenacted, acted out, projected or externalized in relationships and gives rise to destructive and self-destructive motivational forces. Trauma can seep through the layers of culture and society in the manner of toxic chemicals eroding layers of earth. When we look at the "mandala" of trauma in archetypal forms (Wilson, 2003), its presentation includes the vicissitudes of the demonic in its Mephistophelean aspects, expressing the depraved, unholy, sinister, vile and evil elements of the Darkness of Being, which intrusively invade the sanctity of human experiences and the seraphic essence of loving relationships.

Listening to the voices and carefully observing the faces of trauma reveal "snapshots" of the existential struggle to remain whole and vital, and to restore that part of the self scarred by trauma. The stories of trauma survivors are inevitably universal variants of the archetypal abyss of the trauma complex (Wilson, 2003). However, for the psychotherapist, analyst, counselor and others in the helping role, it is the encounter with the voices and faces of the trauma patient that is difficult and painful. Listening empathically to trauma stories is taxing and stressful. It may be illuminating and de-illusioning, compelling soul-searching introspection. To remain sensitive and finely attuned to the internal pain from the individual's psychological injuries requires more than understanding that an experience was traumatic; it requires skill and a capacity to use empathy to access the inner scars of the psyche and the organism itself.

Effective post-traumatic therapy is more than the application of a clinical technique; it is the capacity to facilitate self-healing by helping the patient mobilize and transform the negative energies, memories and emotions of post-traumatic stress disorders (PTSD) and associated conditions into a healthy self-synthesis which evolves into a positive integration of the trauma experience. Therefore the role of a professional therapist entails preparedness for a significant and certain risk of empathic distress, affect dysregulation, compassion fatigue, burnout, countertransference processes and traumatoid states.

THE VOICES AND FACES OF TRAUMA

Listen to the voices of trauma. They are like the top edge of a wave about to break over turbulent ocean water, beneath which lies a potentially deadly rip curl, ready to pull bodies under the surface with a hidden force towards an inexplicable fate.

Trauma Vignettes: Images of the Abyss Experience*

FDNY

"All I could make out was his FDNY badge — *the rest was indescribable —
crushed, burnt remains of a firefighter.*" (Disaster worker, World Trade
Center, 2001, italics ours)

Crushed

"My best friend was crushed underneath a building and asked me for
help, so I tried desperately to help her, but my efforts meant nothing, so I
ran away with another friend. *I hear her voice even now; I'll never be able to
forget it.*" (Hiroshima, 1945, italics ours)

Frozen in Agony

"There were charred dead bodies scattered all over a burned-out field that
once was a residential area. *Bodies frozen in agony reaching up toward the sky.*
Unidentified bodies left like that for days." (Hiroshima, 1945, italics ours)

Childhood in Sarajevo

"God, what have we survived? A beautiful, cultured city in a moment was
transformed into a concentration camp. From surrounding hills, thousands of shells are landing daily. The city is surrounded. For the first
weeks, I took it in with curiosity. *But later, leaving the basement meant death,
when houses around me began to burn, when we began to starve — I understood.*" (Jelacis, age 13, G. White in Figley, 1995, italics ours)

Innocent Brains

"Her [10-year-old] head was injured and *her brain stuck out of her fractured
skull where she hit the hard concrete surface.* Her left eye popped out onto her
cheekbone and blood was coming down her face. She was still alive but
unconscious. I see that at night when I try to go to sleep." (Civil disaster
patient, father of child, 1989, italics ours)

Skinned and Pinned

"We were on search and destroy patrol when we came across his body
[American soldier]. *He had been captured, pinned to a tree and skinned alive.*
His genitals were stuck in his mouth and his eyes were still wide open."
(Vietnam veteran, Bon Song, 1969, italics ours)

Rape Your Children or We Will For You

"I was given another choice: I rape my daughter or the guard does. I tried
to reason with them, telling them that she was an innocent child. I pleaded
with them not to humiliate her, not to hurt her, but instead to *rape me*, to do

---

*Abyss experience is the confrontation with the archetype of trauma: the
demonic, and Darkness of Being (Wilson, 2002, 2003).

with me what they wanted. They laughed and repeated the two choices. I looked at my daughter hoping that she would tell me what to do — our eyes met and I knew that I could not save her from those wretched men. I lowered my eyes in *shame* to keep from seeing my daughter abused. One guard held my face up, forcing me to watch this horrible scene. *I watched, motionless, as she was raped before me and her little brother. When they were through, they forced me to do what they had done to her.* My own daughter, my son forced to watch it all. How could anyone do that? What kind of men are they? What kind of father am I?" (Ortiz, 2001, italics ours)

Human Rain

"It was his last day in Vietnam. He insisted on walking 'point' [first] man. We were near Cambodia — the Black Virgin Mountain area of Tay Ninh. He never saw the command detonated landmine as he stepped on it. *Pieces and parts of his body rained on us — like a shower in blood and pieces of flesh. It smelled horrible. We found what was left of his head and put it in a body bag.*" (Vietnam veteran, Tay Ninh, 1968, italics ours)

Footsteps

"I could tell by my stepfather's footsteps on the wooden hallway floor whether he was drunk when he came down the hallway to my room. When he started in on me [sexual abuse], *I left my body and went away* to a corner of the room, in the ceiling, with my teddy bear." (Sexual abuse victim, 1993, italics ours)

Eyes, Ears, Nose and Mouth

"After the flood stopped, I went over and started taking pieces of wood from the woodpile, and I found a body. I picked up the back of her hair, what hair she had left. She didn't have no clothes on, and *I turned her over and the blood and mud and water came out of her eyes and nose and mouth and ears.* I had to go get clean." (Kai Erikson, Buffalo Creek Dam Disaster, 1974, excerpted, italics ours)

Top Gun in Thailand

"We were on duty in Thailand and received a call that an F-4 Phantom jet was on fire. It landed burning and we [paramedics] responded. We put out the fire and opened the cockpit. The smoke was still pouring out. *I took off the pilots' helmet and blood ran out of his eyes and mouth from his burnt, black face.* He was dead. It was his birthday and he was my best friend. We had planned to party that night." (Vietnam veteran, Thailand, 1968, italics ours)

Frankenstein or Freddy Kruger?

When I woke up after surgery in the burn unit in Japan, they made me look at myself in the mirror. The nurse handed me a mirror and I threw-up [vomited] when I saw the black deformed image that used to be me. I cried for days — it was like looking at a disfigured Halloween mask of a monster." (Vietnam veteran, 1970, Army Burn Unit Hospital, Japan)

Blood on the Tracks
"The Serb snipers were active 24 hours a day. My first hour in Sarajevo, I saw dead bodies on the tram line — women, children and old men — killed in the afternoon — blood on the tramline. What kind of war is this? That was just the beginning for me — everyday some innocent person was killed by a sniper. There were so many killings that they began burying people in the city parks. Bosnia was an evil genocide and the senseless killing has never left me. I still see the blood on the tracks and remember those innocent people." (John P. Wilson, 1994, Sarajevo, italics ours)

Towering Inferno
"I still *hear the screams* and the sounds of the towers collapsing. *I wake up in a sweat, seeing the bodies falling from the tower* — it could have been me — I was on my way to work there [Tower I]. The next day, September 12, 2001, I couldn't feel much of anything. *I was just numb and completely over-whelmed*. New York seemed dead to me. I can still *smell* ground zero in my mind — *it won't ever go away*." (World Trade Center, 2001, italics ours)

Uncle Ho's P.O.W. Crucifixion
"We were forced to watch as he [American P.O.W.] was tortured. They staked him to a pole and broke his bones with a metal rod, starting with his shins. *They inserted a sharp barb-hooked hanger in his belly into his liver and tugged on it until he screamed as if dying*. It was horrible to watch. They shot him slowly, starting with his legs and worked their way up his body, one bullet at a time until the last one killed him … a shot in the forehead. *He had a look of horror in his eyes*. We were forced to watch and warned not to try to escape the camp in Cambodia, where we got caught. He tried to escape and we were given a lesson." (Vietnam veteran, 1970, italics ours)

No Limits to Marquis de Sade
"During his first arrest 'L' tried to commit suicide, but he was shot in the leg and taken directly to a notorious prison. There he was immediately beaten brutally over his entire body, hooded, and subjected to falanga [beating the soles of the feet]. The torture continued and 'L' was forced to lick up blood from the floor. He was suspended on a cross, kicked over his entire body, and kept awake for days. Not broken by the physical torture, 'L' was sub-jected to psychological torture. He was placed in a room between a mother and a daughter. The mother was whipped and ordered not to make a sound or the daughter would be abused. He was subjected to mock execution sev-eral times; on one such occasion he was drenched with litres of petrol, and the torturers fumbled with matches in front of him. Threatened with homosexual rape and beaten to unconsciousness, he also received electrical

torture around the ears. His nose was broken repeatedly, and he developed bleeding from the stomach and hemorrhagic vomiting. He was suspended both head up and feet up, and burned with cigarettes over his body. He could exhibit a multitude of scars from these burns. Subsequently, 'L' was isolated for about a year in a very small, completely barren cell. In this new prison he was also subjected to Russian roulette and deprivation of food. Later because of gangrene of the feet he was taken to a hospital outside the prison, and there he managed to escape." (Torture victim, RCT, 1992)

Saigon Refugee and Asylum Seeker
"I was captured before the end of the war in Saigon in 1975. As an officer of the Vietnam Army, I was taken North with other P.O.W.s who were offi- cers. We were put into bamboo cages … Everyday we were spread eagled on a flat table and tortured. They would ask questions and burn our skin, nipples, and face with cigarettes … I ran away one night and escaped. I came to the U.S. seeking asylum in Cleveland, Ohio. I dream of these experiences even today." (Vietnam refugee, 2002)

Hippocrates Incurable Vivisection in Living Color
"Cannibalism and vivisection of allied flyers by the Japanese is quite well documented. Kyushi Imperial University officials, for example, have acknowledged vivisecting eight [U.S.] B-29 crewmen in experiments car- ried out on May 17, 23, 29 and June 3, 1945. In one experiment, [Dr.] Ishiyama extracted an American P.O.W.'s lungs and placed them in a sur- gical pan. He made an incision in the lung artery and allowed blood to flow into the chest cavity, killing the man. In another experiment, Ishiyama removed a prisoner's stomach, then cut five ribs and held a large artery near the heart to determine how long he could stop the blood flow before the victim died. In a third, another Japanese doctor made four openings in a prisoner's skull and inserted a knife into the brain to see what the reaction would be. The prisoner died." (Ienaga, 1968)

As we read these vignettes, they evoke our own associations, images, feelings and attempts to frame a context and perspective of understand- ing. Each voice is unique, real and a part of history, past and present. These authentic vignettes are only excerpts of much more detailed trauma stories of some of our patients and other survivors of massive, cata- strophic trauma. Metaphorically, they are like the top edge of a wave breaking over the surf. The trauma therapist must "flow" with the wave or risk the overpowering currents of the rip curl beneath the surface.

THE TRANSMITTING UNCONSCIOUS OF TRAUMATIZATION

Trauma work challenges the therapist's or professional's capacity to be empathic and effective when working with clients who suffer from PTSD.

Seeing the faces of trauma clients and listening to their voices and their individual stories is a form of traumatic encounter in itself which has been called secondary traumatization (Stamm, 1997), vicarious traumatization (Pearlman & Saativne, 1995), compassion fatigue (Figley, 1995), empathic strain (Wilson & Lindy, 1994), trauma-related affective reactions (ARs; Wilson & Lindy, 1994) and trauma-related countertransference processes. In this book, we will refer to such reactions as *traumatoid states*, a form of occupational stress which results from work with trauma victims.

Trauma work requires the therapist's immersion into the phenomenal reality and ego-space of the person suffering from PTSD. *Empathic attunement* is the capacity to resonate efficiently and accurately to another's state of being; to match self–other understanding; to have knowledge of the internal psychological ego-states of another who has suffered a trauma; and to understand the unique internal working model/schema of their trauma experience. Empathic capacity is the aptitude for empathic attunement, and varies greatly among therapists working with PTSD patients (Dalenberg, 2000). Effective post-traumatic therapy rests on the cornerstone of empathic ability and the facility to sustain empathic attunement. Empathic capacity is a fundamental dimension of the psychobiology of empathy. In a clinical setting, a good therapist has the ability to "decode" trauma stories and *trauma specific transference* (TST) reactions — those that emanate from the client and are transmitted to the therapist in multiple channels of communication (Wilson & Lindy, 1994).

Empathic attunement is part of the process of decoding, a *signal detection* process of information flowing from the patient (sender) to the therapist who, in some basic respects, serves as a "radio" or "satellite" receiver who hones in on a signal being transmitted and decodes its message. Indeed, it is entirely possible to speak of TST reactions, the disclosure of the trauma story, and the flow of affect, cognition and behavior (including especially nonverbal actions), as multichanneled messages being sent from the patient to the therapist. If visualized, one would see patterns or images of energy in wave form emanating from the trauma client and manifesting themselves in various amplitudes and frequencies as they flow in patterns towards the receptor site of the therapist's mind and consciousness. To adequately receive and decode the message without *noise* or *interference*, the therapist must have a capacity for decoding, interpreting and responding with information to the client as part of the interactional communication sequence (Tansey & Burke, 1989). Viewing these processes historically, Freud used a similar metaphor in one of his few writings on countertransference. In a paper written in 1912 to general medical practitioners, he stated,

> To put it into a formula: [the therapist] must turn his own unconscious like a receptive organ toward the transmitting unconscious of the patient. He

must adjust himself to the patient as a telephone receiver is adjusted to the transmitting microphone. Just as the receiver converts back into sound waves the electric oscillations ... so the doctor's unconscious is able, from the derivation of the unconscious which is communicated to him, to reconstruct the unconscious, which has determined the patient's free associations. (italics ours; pp. 111–120)

Freud understood that the interactional communication sequence in treatment was dynamic in nature, and involved both the patient's *and* the therapist's unconscious processes. However, he did not elaborate on the mechanisms of countertransference in detail. In his widely cited 1910 paper, Freud stated that it was critical for the analyst to

recognize this counter-transference in himself and overcome it ... we have noticed that no psychoanalyst goes further than his own complexes and resistances permit, and we consequently require that he shall begin activity with a self-analysis and continually carry it deeper while he is making his own observations on his patients. Anyone who fails to produce results in a self-analysis of this kind may at once give up any idea of being able to treat patients by analysis. (pp. 141–142)

This passage illustrates that Freud believed that a therapist's self-knowledge of how his own unconscious thought processes were activated "by the transmitting unconscious of the patient" was central to successful treatment. We can view the role of empathy as central to post-traumatic therapy; it is a vehicle to portals of entry into the interior space of the psyche. Like the ancient pyramids, the ego has secret passageways into inner sanctums, burial tombs, rooms and chambers which are rich in artifacts and valued objects of practical and symbolic significance. For patients with PTSD, these tombs are often horror chambers filled with traumatic memories and emotions of terror, dread, fear and the confrontation with the abyss of darkness which has been sealed over and buried. In some cases, the hidden chambers are carefully sealed in darkness and not meant to be discovered.

Empathy is the psychological capacity to identify and understand another person's psychological state of being (Wilson & Lindy, 1994). Empathic attunement allows access to the passageway and portals of the ego's "pyramid." As defined fundamentally by Kohut (1959, 1977), empathy is a form of "knowing," information processing and "data collection" about another or what is referred to as a *self-object*. Rowe and MacIsaac (1991) state that "empathic immersion into the patient's experience focuses the analyst's attention upon what it is like to be the subject rather than the target of the patient's wishes and demands" (p. 18). Similarly, they note that "the empathic process is employed solely as a scientific tool to enable the analyst eventually to make interpretations to the patient that are as accurate and complete as possible" (p. 64). We can view empathy, then, as the primary tool for accessing the ego-state of the patient suffering from PTSD. Slatker (1987), in a review of empathy in analytic theory, states,

> empathy is based on counter-identification; indeed, it is counter-identification that permits our empathy to be therapeutically useful ... the analyst's negative counter-transferential reactions can cause his empathy to diminish or even vanish altogether. When this happens, he may become vulnerable to additional negative counter-transference reactions. (p. 203)

The patient's ego-state or ego-spatial configuration includes the organization of experience into memory which governs attempts at adaptation to self, others and the world. It represents the fluctuating dimensions of self-reference which includes cognitive functions, affect regulation, ego-identity and a sense of well-being (Schore, 2003b; Wilson, Friedman, & Lindy, 2001). Moreover, at least five portals of entry into the ego-states of the PTSD client are pathways created by PTSD symptoms, which are organized into five clusters within the organism (i.e., PTSD: [1] reexperiencing, [2] avoidance, [3] hyperarousal, [4] ego-identity self-processes and [5] interpersonal attachment) (Wilson, Friedman, & Lindy, 2001). These five portals of entry give the therapist an insight into an understanding of the different symptom channels or manifestations that comprise the information transmission being generated in specific forms of transference during treatment. Empathy, as one method of connecting to the ego-state and the unconscious process of the trauma client, allows the therapist to creatively attune to five different PTSD channels of information transmission being generated by the patient.

INFORMATION TRANSMISSION OR FLOW IN THE TRANSFERENCE–COUNTER-TRANSFERENCE MATRIX

When the patient and therapist are together in the safety of the clinician's office, information is exchanged during the treatment. To an outside observer, not much appears to be happening apart from a verbal exchange for a brief period of time. Indeed, if videotaped and presented to viewers without sound content, it would appear that the two people seated across the desk could be talking anywhere — for example, at a restaurant, in a living room, in a hotel lobby, or in a business office. Indeed, Freud (1917) made a similar observation about the process of psychoanalysis:

> Nothing takes place in a psychoanalytic treatment but an interchange of words between the patient and the analyst. The patient talks, tells of his past experiences and present impressions, complains, confesses to his wishes and his emotional impulses. The doctor listens, tries to direct the patient's processes of thought, exhorts, forces his attention in certain directions, gives him explanations and observes the reactions of understanding or rejection which he [the doctor] in this way provokes in him. (pp. 19, 20)

Freud's observation about an exchange of words, and the role of the analyst as one who gently guides the conversation and the use of free association, is instructive. It depicts the therapist as one who observes, gathers information, and probes into different areas of the patient's past history. Freud's (1912) work makes it evident that he understood that the therapist must use his "unconscious" as a "receptive organ" to the "transmitting unconscious of the patient." The process of dynamic interchange between the patient and the analyst involves *unconscious* and *conscious* reception of information. In other words, *there are multiple channels of information being transmitted by the patient*: (1) words, (2) affects, (3) memories, (4) thoughts, (5) body postures, (6) voice modulations, (7) expressions of personality and (8) "here and now" ego-state presentations of the saliency of integrative consciousness during a period of time. These dimensions of the patient, in the context of a therapeutic relationship, can be meaningfully thought of as forms of information transmission about the patient's individual dynamics. *They are transference projections or transmissions of psychological functioning. The transmissions of data are different types of information flow emanating from the patient through encoded channels.* Figure 1.1 illustrates these mechanisms and reveals that the patient (sender) transmits information flow in a variety of forms, including transference dynamics. The therapist (receiver) is the object of the patient's information transmission, and attempts clinically to decode the information encoded in the different channels.

If we consider post-traumatic therapy as an active process, terms such as *flow, wave, signal, energy, transmission* and *information gathering* may be used to characterize the nature of the transmitting unconscious of the patient. These defining concepts illustrate the features of a multichanneled process of verbal and nonverbal information transmission (earlier referred to as TST) which vary in their *intensity, frequency, amplitude* and *modulation* in each channel of information transmission. In this regard, it is possible to conceptualize that, at any given time, seven separate channels transmit to the therapist (affect, defense, somatic state, ego-state, personality, unconscious memory and cognitive processes). These same seven channels exist as potential receptor sites in the therapist. In a manner similar to a neuron, information flows, or is transmitted, from one part of the nerve across a synapse to an awaiting receptor location which receives the transmission, decodes it and activates another process. In essence then, encoded information is transmitted, decoded and capable of being processed for use in the treatment process. When construed in this way, it becomes evident that empathic attunement is a vehicle for accurate reception of the information being generated by the patient. Therapeutic effectiveness requires accurate decoding of the channels, and the ability and capacity to hold (i.e., store) the information without overloading the capacities of the therapist channels (system overload). Transference and countertransference are clinical terms,

"The transmitting unconscious of the patient" (Freud, 1912)

Defining Concepts: Flow, Energy, Transmission, Waves, Information, Channels, Signal Sending, Somatic Processes, Unconscious Projection

Features: Multichannel Processes of Verbal, Nonverbal and Somatic Information Transmission

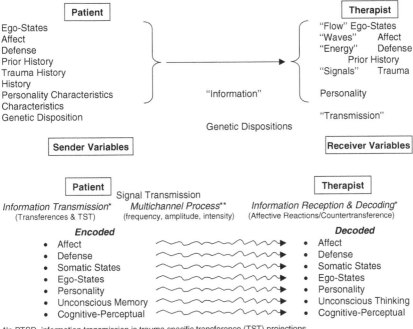

Figure 1.1 Information flow in the transference–counter-transference matrix. Copyright John P. Wilson, 2002.

rooted in psychoanalysis, to describe the intricate and extraordinarily interesting process of human communication in the context of psychotherapy.

TRAUMA SPECIFIC TRANSFERENCE TRANSMISSIONS: ORGANISMIC PROJECTIONS OF EMBEDDED PSYCHIC TRAUMA

Figure 1.2 illustrates how PTSD symptoms get transmitted during the process of psychotherapy. It is especially important to understand TST since it is always present during the treatment, prior to resolution and integration of the trauma experience. It is our belief, clinically demonstrable in training work, that TST is composed of a set of cues that are "leaked" out in subtle expressions in the seven channels shown in

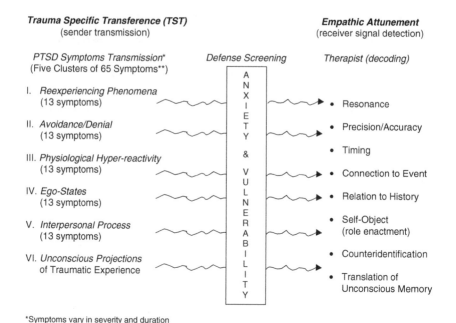

Figure 1.2 Trauma specific transference transmission (TSTT). Copyright John P. Wilson, 2002.

Figure 1.1. More specifically, there are at least 65 distinct symptoms of PTSD (Wilson, Friedman, & Lindy, 2001), as well as unconscious projections of the trauma experience across the five clusters of PTSD symptoms: (1) reexperiencing, (2) avoidance/denial, (3) psychological hyper-reactivity, (4) ego-state, and (5) interpersonal process. In this regard, one may consider TST as omnipresent. It is as if the victim speaks out: "See what happened to me. Look at what the trauma did to change the way I used to be." *Thus, TST is an unconscious ego-state projection of the entire organism's response to traumatization and the changes induced at all levels of psychological functioning* (i.e., allostatic changes; see chapter 11 for a discussion). Further, the unconscious is a kind of "diplomatic spokesperson" who conveys messages to the therapist in this information transmission via the seven channels. Unconscious projections require decoding and understanding; they are behavioral manifestations, sometimes symbolic, of that which the patient cannot express or recall by conscious effort.

CASE EXAMPLE: MASHED BRAINS AT DAWN

A Vietnam War veteran patient used to pick at the soles of his boots with a pencil as he talked, for years, about his overwhelming combat experiences. With a sad, tired, forlorn expression on his prematurely aged face, he would repeatedly say, "You know, doc, there is something missing about that night-long firefight." As it turned out, the soldier's unconscious picking at his boots with a pencil was a reenactment of the gruesome experience of using a stick to pick out, from the cleats in his boots, the mashed brains of one of his buddies who died in the night-long firefight in which all but three platoon members were killed. This action of picking at his boots during treatment is a clear example of trauma specific transference transmission (TSTT) and a reenactment of the original post-combat reaction. It was as if his unconscious voice was transmitting the message: "Look here, doc, here is the clue to what I can't remember." Indeed, when his amnesia dissipated, he recalled the entire forgotten sequence of events of the night battle which, as a 19-year-old soldier in the 196th Light Infantry Brigade, changed his life forever. The terror, fear of annihilation and immersion into human carnage was devastating to his ego and his capacity to master the experience. He always remembered sitting on a log, picking at the gray brain matter in the morning at "first light," as the sun broke through rain clouds and morning mist, in the mountains of the central highlands of Vietnam in 1967. His life changed forever on that day.

The image of a young soldier sitting alone, battle weary and totally exhausted, picking human brains from the sole of his battle-worn combat boots, encapsulated his current reality of being alone, divorced, isolated, alienated from others and depressed. For him, the memories of war were his link to the past, buddies killed and his search for meaning. The unintegrated memories were bittersweet companions: they tortured him and sustained him at the same time. His unconscious fear was that if he let go of the most powerful experience of his life, he would be letting go of himself and his identity. The question for him, of course, centered around the issue of "What's left, doc?" In other words, he was "picking" at the meaning of his life after Vietnam.

EMPATHIC ATTUNEMENT AND DECODING TRAUMA SPECIFIC TRANSFERENCE

The magnitude and power of the complexity of TSTT cannot be underestimated in the treatment of PTSD. It is one of the critically important features that differentiate PTSD treatment from that of therapeutic approaches to other psychiatric disorders, including anxiety disorders. The clinician's ability to decode TSTT will be strongly associated with therapeutic outcome. Viewed in this way, the central role of empathic attunement takes on a clearer focus, since it is a primary clinical skill for entering one of the "pyramidal" portals into the PTSD patient's ego-state. Conceptually, however, there is an advantage in this perspective, since awareness of the seven channels of information for the five clusters of PTSD symptoms allows the therapist ways of *knowing* and approaching how to decode the TSTT and other transmissions. Recognition of the universality of unconscious projections of the traumatic experience in any of the seven channels of the PTSD symptoms enables the therapist to formulate hypotheses and informed intuitions about the meaning and significance of any interactional sequence during treatment. In this regard, it is our belief that there is no randomness in the patterns of TSTT; they have meaning and significance at all times.

Moreover, as Figure 1.2 illustrates, ego-defenses serve as *screens, filters, blocks* and control mechanisms to TSTT. The various defenses are control mechanisms directly concerned with anxiety and states of vulnerability. The greater the experienced (conscious or unconscious) anxiety and inner vulnerability, the more the defenses will be utilized to stave off threats (i.e., reexperienced traumatic memories) which were originally embedded in the trauma experience, or which activate prior emotional trauma or conflicts from the patient's history.

However, we wish to emphasize that what we are proposing is not the classic Freudian paradigm of trauma and defense against traumatic anxiety (Freud, 1917, 1920). Rather, it is a paradigm in which allostatic transformations, caused by trauma, alter organismic functioning in a holistic, dynamic manner (see chapter 11). These alterations, produced by trauma, impact all levels of psychological functioning in synergistic ways. The organismic impacts are dynamically interrelated and express themselves in various channels of transmission and behavior. Traumatic encoding of experience is organismic; it is not an isolated subsystem of memory, affect, perception or motivation. TSTT are direct manifestations of this set of organismic changes caused by trauma. Traumatic experiences, by definition, are forms of extreme stress with varying degrees of power to energize the organism's functioning and disrupt natural states of well-being. Traumatic experiences are not the same as normal developmental life experiences or hassles; they are beyond the line demarcating *usual* and *normal* from *unusual* and *abnormal*. Extreme trauma, especially catastrophic trauma involving the abyss experience (Wilson, 2003), can be thought of as "Big Bang" phenomena, in a manner akin to the Big Bang theory of the universe. The Big Bang of profoundly catastrophic trauma can rattle the organism to the core, rearranging its essential form without destroying it completely. The result of the post-traumatic *shake up* to organismic functioning is allostatic transformations of energy, which now have a *program* and a *life force* of their own until treatment and healing restores organismic well-being, albeit in a different structural configuration from that which existed prior to the shattering caused by the trauma experience.

REFERENCES

Dalenberg, C. L. (2000). *Countertransference and PTSD*. Washington, DC: American Psychological Association Press.

Danieli, Y. (1988). Confronting the unimaginable: Psychotherapists' reactions to victims of the Nazi Holocaust. In J. P. Wilson, Z. Harel, & B. Kahana (Eds.), *Human adaptation to extreme stress* (pp. 219–237). New York: Plenum Press.

Figley, C. R. (1995). *Compassion fatigue*. New York: Brunner/Mazel.

Figley, C. R. (2002). *Treating compassion fatigue*. New York: Brunner-Routledge.

Freud, S. (1910). The future prospects of psychoanalytic therapy. In J. Strachey (Ed. & Trans.), *The standard edition of the complete psychological works of Sigmund Freud* (Vol. 11, pp. 141–142). London: Hogarth Press.

Freud, S. (1912). Recommendations to physicians practicing psychoanalysis. In *The standard edition of the complete psychological works of Sigmund Freud* (Vol. 12, pp. 111–120). London: Hogarth Press.

Freud, S. (1917). *New introductory lectures on psychoanalysis*. New York: Norton.

Freud, S. (1917). *Introductory lecture on psychoanalysis*. New York: Norton.

Freud, S. (1928). *Beyond the pleasure principle*. New York: Norton.

Jung, C. G. (1929). The therapeutic value of abreaction (H. Read, M. Fordham, & G. Adler, Eds., Vol. 16). In *Collected works of C. J. Jung* (Vols. 1–20, R. F. C. Hull, Trans.). Princeton, NJ: Princeton University Press.

Kohut, H. (1959). Introspection, empathy and psychoanalysis. *Journal of American Psychoanalytic Association, 7,* 459–483.

Kohut, H. (1977). *The restoration of the self*. New York: International Universities Press.

Lifton, R. J. (1967). *Death in life: The survivors of Hiroshima*. New York: Simon & Schuster.

Lifton, R. J. (1993). From Hiroshima to the Nazi doctors: The evolution of psychoformative approaches to understanding traumatic stress syndromes. In J. P. Wilson & B. Raphael (Eds.), *International handbook of traumatic stress syndromes* (pp. 11–25). New York: Plenum Press.

Ortiz, D. (2001). The survivor perspective: Voices from the center. In E. Gerrity, T. M. Keane, & F. Tuma (Eds.), *Mental health consequences of torture* (pp. 3–13). New York: Kluwer/Plenum Press.

Pearlman, L. & Saakvitne, K. (1995). *Trauma and the therapist*. New York: Norton.

Rowe, T. & MacIsaac, J. (1991). *Empathic attunement*. Northvale, NJ: Jason Aronson.

Schore, A. N. (2003a). *Affect dysregulation and disorders of the self*. New York: Norton.

Schore, A. N. (2003b). *Affect regulation and the repair of the self*. New York: Norton.

Slatker, E. (1987). *Countertransference*. Northvale, NJ: Jason Aronson.

Stamm, B. H. (1997). *Secondary traumatic stress*. Lutherville, MD: Sidran Press.

Stamm, B. H. (1999). *Secondary traumatic stress: Self-care for clinicians, researchers and educators*. Cutherville, MD: Sidran Press.

Tansey, M. J. & Burke, W. F. (1989). *Understanding countertransference*. Hillsdale, NJ: Erlbaum.

Wilson, J. P. (2002, October). *The abyss experience and catastrophic stress*. Presentation at St. Joseph's University, Terrorism and Weapons of Mass Destruction, Philadelphia, PA.

Wilson, J. P. (2003). *Empathic strain and post-traumatic therapy*. New York: Guilford Publications.

Wilson, J. P. (2004). Broken spirits. In J. P. Wilson & B. Drozdek (Eds.), *Broken spirits: The treatment of traumatized asylum seekers, refugees and war and torture victims* (pp. 141–173). New York: Brunner-Routledge.

Wilson, J. P., Friedman, M. J. & Lindy, J. D. (2001). *Treating psychological trauma and PTSD*. New York: Guilford Publications.

Wilson, J. & Lindy, J. (1994). *Countertransference in the treatment of PTSD*. New York: Guilford Publications.

2

The Matrix of Empathy

Empathy ... is the capacity to think and feel oneself into the inner life of another person.

The Analysis of the Self (H. Kohut, 1971, p. 82)

The nature of empathy in the treatment of traumatized states is a richly complex matrix. As a psychobiological capacity, empathy is embedded within the organism, shaped by early attachment experiences (Eisenberg, Murphy, & Shepard, 1997) and refined by social learning, personal experience, personality and moral development (Aronoff & Wilson, 1985; Staub, 1979).

In treatment for post-traumatic stress disorder (PTSD) and the sequelae of traumatic injuries, therapists respond instinctively and intuitively to the levels of clients' pain, direct distress or sealed-over psychic numbing. Therapists aim to sustain a centered focus by drawing on their own experiences with pain, uncertainty, anxiety, suffering and memories of profoundly upsetting life experiences in an attempt to understand the client's inner struggles with psychic trauma and how it has altered their world and reality. The therapist attempts to match understanding of the client's internal state and to empathically "walk where they walked" in order to know more precisely the intricacies of the client's trauma experience.

The purpose of this chapter is to present the matrix of trauma and the relevant concepts that will form the theoretical and clinical framework of this book. To do so requires clarification on the objectives, purposes and diversity of concepts utilized in developing the ideas that will be presented with regard to the nature of empathy in the treatment of trauma and PTSD.

The primary purpose of this book is to explore the central role of empathy in the treatment of trauma victims. Our analysis of empathy extends to all victims of physical and psychological trauma, not just persons suffering from PTSD. We believe that there are universal effects of trauma and states of traumatization which reflect the specific types of injury to the mind and body. As the ancient Greeks understood, trauma inflicts wounds and injuries to previously intact states of being, resulting in traumatized states. The word *traumatization* refers to changes in functioning produced by an externally inflicted injury. To understand states of traumatization requires empathy with and knowledge of the nature of the wounds and injuries inflicted by the forces of nature or by humankind. Empathy, as noted by Kohut (1971), is a means of knowing what it is like to be the subject, rather than the object, of inquiry. Empathy, as a psychobiological capacity, is a means of entering the phenomenal reality of the trauma victim to understand the internal working schema of the trauma experience and its effects on intrapsychic processes. Empathy, then, is also a means of knowledge acquisition and a tool of discovery of the trauma patient's inner world. It is a process of discovering the nature of the trauma landscape which characterizes alter states of well-being.

To illustrate how empathy "works" in the treatment of states of traumatization and PTSD, we will develop a conceptual model of empathy as a psychological process. This model is generic in nature, and potentially generalizable to other areas of psychological study beyond understanding empathic processes in relation to psychological trauma (i.e. social psychology, altruism, prosocial behavior, group dynamics, medical diagnosis, etc.).

Our focus on empathy will require consideration of a wide range of questions. For example: How does empathy influence such processes as the development of a therapeutic alliance, trust and the patient's willingness to fully disclose the most difficult aspects of personal abuse or the specific details of an overwhelming trauma experience? How does empathy affect the nature and dynamics of transference and countertransference during the treatment process? How does empathy affect the ability to accurately make proper diagnoses of psychiatric disorders? How does empathy affect the structure and process of psychotherapy and influence the success or failure of outcomes? How does empathy relate to the repeated exposure of therapists to stressful encounters with trauma clients and the disposition to experience compassion fatigue, vicarious traumatization, secondary traumatic stress and empathic strain? How does empathy play a role in the onset of traumatoid states, an inclusive term which, we will suggest, encompasses the current understanding of occupationally related stress response syndromes (OSRS)? Finally, how does empathy relate to the transformation of trauma? Are there states of "high empathic" functioning which facilitate the processing, assimilation and resolution of PTSD and states of traumatization? If so, what are the personality and behavioral characteristics of the "high empathy therapist?" All these questions are examined in the chapters that follow.

THE NATURE OF EMPATHY

The matrix of empathy comprises interacting and intersecting psychological processes which include affect, cognition, perception, communication processes, interpersonal styles, modalities of empathic attunement and

strain, personality characteristics, dyadic interactions, transference–
countertransference processes, the operation of security and defensive
mechanisms, and knowledge of the dynamics of post-traumatic states.
The matrix also has specific anchor points in conceptual terminology
which reflect the rapid growth of research and scientific knowledge in the
field of traumatology. The nomenclature of traumatic events are terms of
art, clinical phenomenology and empirical science which have evolved
along somewhat parallel courses as the knowledge base of PTSD and
traumatoid states has expanded worldwide in scope (see Wilson,
Friedman, & Lindy, 2001, for a discussion). The rapid growth in new
information, psychological/psychiatric terms and scientific findings on
PTSD and trauma requires the creation of a glossary to define the terms
that will be used throughout this book. Figure 2.1 presents, in alphabeti-
cal order, the terms that the reader can reference as needed.

Abyss Experience – Individual encounters with extremely foreboding psychological
experience, which typically involve the confrontation with evil and death; the experience
of soul death and the specter of nonbeing; the sense of abandonment by humanity; the
sense of ultimate aloneness in the universe and despairing; and the cosmic challenge
of meaning

Affect Dysregulation – The change in normal capacity for regulating emotional states; a
characteristic of prolonged stress response in PTSD

Affective Reaction (AR) – The experience of affect by the therapist in response to
transference reaction by the client

Allostasis – Resetting the baseline of physiological/psychological functioning following
traumatic experience; allostasis is differentiated from homeostasis, or the tendency to
seek equilibrium in system functioning; allostasis is characterized by stability through
changed homeostatic functioning

Anxiety and Defensiveness in Post-traumatic Therapy – The commonly experienced
states of anxiety, tension, irritability, fear, uncertainty, anger, etc. which are indigenous to
post-traumatic therapies; the symptoms of anxiety and defensiveness in post-traumatic
therapies reflect Type I and Type II countertransference processes, empathic strain and
empathic rupture

Archetype of Trauma – Universal forms of trauma experience present in all cultures and
having personal and historical significance; the Trauma Archetype is related to the formation of the Trauma Complex (Wilson, 2002, 2003, 2004)

Clinicians' Trauma Reaction Survey – A questionnaire developed to assess empathic
strains and countertransference reactions in the course of post-traumatic therapy

Compassion Fatigue – A term that "can be used interchangeably by those who feel
uncomfortable with STS and STSD" (Figley, 1995), compassion fatigue is the stress
and strain of caring for others who are ill or suffering due to medical illness or psychological maladies

---

Figure 2.1 Glossary of terms relevant to empathy in the treatment of trauma and PTSD.

Counteridentification – The process by which the therapist attempts to maintain objectivity in treatment by examining his or her identification with the client in an empathic role stance

Countertransference Reactions (CTRs) – The therapist's affective, somatic, cognitive and interpersonal reactions (including defensive) toward the client's story and behaviors

Determinants of Countertransference Processes – The four categorical determinants typically associated with the onset of empathic strains and the development of countertransference processes: (1) trauma history of client; (2) therapist's personality processes and defenses; (3) client's idiosyncratic personality processes; (4) organizational/institutional climate

Dimensions of Empathic Functioning – The psychological dimensions of empathic functioning, which include capacity, resistance, tolerance and sensitivity, and endurance

Dual Countertransference – CTRs toward two or more objects at the same time (e.g., a client and an institution where therapist is employed)

Dual Unfolding Process – The evolving nature of the transference–countertransference process in the course of treatment

Dyschronicity – Response mismatching or ineffectiveness in the communication process between therapist and client

Empathic Attunement – The psychobiological capacity to experience, understand and communicate knowledge of the internal psychological state of being of another person. Empathic attunement is characterized by accurate emotional resonance, synchrony, the ability to decode multichanneled signal transmissions (e.g., nonverbal, emotional, physical/somatic states, cognitive processes, ego-defenses, ego-states, etc.) from another person and manifest coetaneous matching responses which are experienced by the recipients as being understood, "in phase" and "on target" with what they were sending as communications of information about their psychological processes (Wilson, 2003)

Empathic Balance Beam – The processes of attempting to maintain balance between modes of empathic attunement and modes of empathic strain

Empathic Behavioral Enactment – The behavioral disposition to manifest empathic functioning in the continuum of empathic processes

Empathic Continuum – A continuum of degrees of empathic functioning which ranges from minimal empathy (detachment, separation, absence) to maximum empathic functioning (engagement, attunement, presence)

Empathic Identification – The processes of identifying with the internal psychological state of another person

Empathic Rupture – The rupture in the quality of empathic attunement which may result in loss of therapeutic alliance and pathogenic consequences for the patient's progress and recovery during treatment

Figure 2.1 (continued)

Empathic Strain – Interpersonal or other factors significantly affecting the capacity for sustained empathic attunement and resulting in loss of capacity for resonance, synchrony, congruence in communication with stress; in psychotherapy and work with trauma patients, empathic strain refers to factors in the therapist, in the patient or in dyadic interaction that impair or limit or adversely impact the therapeutic process (Wilson, 2003)

Empathic Stretch – The capacity of therapists to stretch beyond their usual limits to achieve resonant empathic response with clients

Empathy – The psychobiological capacity to express another person's state of being and phenomenological perspective at any given moment in time

Factors Determining Empathic Orientation – The primary factors determining a person's empathic orientation, which include developmental socialization, ego-maturity, trauma history, life experience, and attachment capacity

High Empathic Capacity – The personality characteristic of the highly empathic person who exhibits cross-situational consistency in empathic functioning; characteristics include optimal attunement, good signal detection and decoding ability, good affect modulation, good cadence and timing of responsiveness, phasic continuity and altruism

Hyperarousal – Excessive autonomic nervous system reactivity as a manifestation of acute, prolonged or chronic stress response syndromes

Internal Working Model or Schema – A term used to describe the nature of a patient's inner world of psychological functioning, including drives, conflicts, defenses and states of traumatization

Isochronicity – Response matching in the communication process between therapist and client

Modes of Empathic Attunement – The primary modes of manifesting empathic attunement in the processes of psychotherapy, which include empathic strength, empathic accuracy, empathic inconsistency, empathic weakness, empathic distancing and empathic insufficiency

Modes of Empathic Strain – The primary modes of manifesting empathic strain, which include empathic disequilibrium, empathic withdrawal, empathic enmeshment and empathic repression

Objective CTRs – Expectable and indigenous ARs by the therapist during the course of treatment

Occupational Stress Response Syndromes (OSRS) – A pattern of prolonged occupationally related stress response syndromes that develop following exposure to stressful and often repetitive demands associated with work responsibilities.

Organismic Embedding of Trauma – The multisystem encoding and embedding of traumatic experiences within the organism

Positive Allostasis – The transformation of allostatically disrupted systems of functioning and adaptation into optimal, positive levels of functioning and adaptation

Figure 2.1 (continued)

PTSD Triad – The three primary symptom clusters of PTSD: (1) reexperiencing trauma (traumatic memory); (2) avoidance, numbing and defensive patterns; and (3) hyper-arousal states and changes in the psychobiology of stress response

Qualities of Empathic Attunement – The psychological dimensions underlying the quality of empathic responding, which include resonance, intensity, timing, accuracy, prediction and isochronicity

Safe-Holding Environment – D. W. Winnicott's term for a therapeutic context that is perceived by the client as a safe, protective environment which can successfully contain or hold the client's emotional difficulties that led to treatment

Secondary Traumatic Stress (STS) – "The natural consequent behaviors and emotions resulting from knowing about a traumatizing event experienced by a significant other — the stress resulting from helping or wanting to help a traumatized or suffering person" (Figley, 1993,1995)

Secondary Traumatic Stress Disorder (STSD) – "STSD is a syndrome of symptoms nearly identical to PTSD, except that exposure to knowledge about a traumatizing event experienced by a significant other is associated with a set of STSD symptoms, and PTSD symptoms are directly connected to the sufferer, the person suffering from primary traumatic stress" (Figley, 1995)

Signal Detection of Trauma Symptoms – The ability to detect symptoms transmitted by patients with a significant history of trauma; the signals are trauma specific and encoded with seven primary channels reflecting the organismic embedding of the trauma experience

Subjective CTRs – ARs manifested by the therapist to the transference that are idiosyncratic and particular and may involve personal conflicts that are unresolved

Sustained Empathic Inquiry – The therapist's capacity to remain in an empathic role stance toward the client throughout the course of treatment

Synergistic Interaction – Reciprocal and multiple determinants of stress response systems within the organism, especially in respect of traumatic states

Tetrahedral Model of PTSD and Dissociation – A three-dimensional model of PTSD as a system, developed by Wilson, Friedman, and Lindy (2001), which includes the diagnostic clusters of PTSD and impairments in self-capacities and attachment relationship; the post-traumatic symptom clusters are encapsulated in a tetrahedral model which also extends to dissociative processes

Transference – The process and behaviors by which a client relates to the therapist in a manner similar to that in past relationships with significant others

Transference Projections – Projective processes externalized by the patient and projected into the therapeutic relationship

Transference Themes and Encoded Memories – Ten universal transference themes associated with trauma specific transference (TST) which encode memories and affects of the trauma experience

Figure 2.1 (continued)

Transmitting Unconscious Process – The transmission of unconscious mental processes in seven channels: (1) affect; (2) defense; (3) somatic states; (4) ego-states; (5) personality processes; (6) cognitive-perceptual processes; and (7) unconscious memory (implicit memory systems)

Trauma Complex – A complex of symptoms, behavioral dispositions and intrapsychic processes which develop after trauma; the 10 dimensions of the Trauma Complex include PTSD symptoms and intrapsychic processes involving the self and personal identity configurations (Wilson, 2003, 2004)

Trauma Decoding – The process of decoding trauma specific transference and trauma specific transmissions of data sent in the seven primary channels of transmission (see Trauma Specific Transference)

Trauma Specific Transference (TST) – Transference reactions specifically associated with unmetabolized elements of the traumatic event and usually involving symbolic and other forces of reenactment with the therapist

Trauma Specific Trauma Transference (TSTT) – The transmission of trauma and PTSD-related information either in conscious or unconscious forms, through the seven primary channels of transmission (see Transmitting Unconscious Process)

Trauma Story – The trauma survivor's account of his or her experience in a traumatic event

Traumatoid States – The psychological reactions of professionals and others who work with victims of trauma. Traumatoid states are trauma-like reactions that develop after significant exposure to a traumatized person and include symptoms of dysregulated affects, somatic reactions, hyperarousal, and tendencies to reexperience or avoid the traumatized person's report of his or her physical or psychological injuries which were not present before such experiences

Type I CTRs – CTRs that involve forms of denial, detachment, distancing or withdrawal from the client

Type II CTRs – CTRs that involve forms of overidentification, enmeshment or overidealization of the client

Vicarious Traumatization (VT) – "Vicarious traumatization refers to a transformation in the therapist's (or other trauma worker's) inner experience resulting from empathic engagement with the client's trauma material. That is, through exposure to clients' graphic accounts of sexual abuse experiences and to the realities of people's intentional cruelty to one another, and through the inevitable re-enactments in the therapy relationship, the therapist is vulnerable through his or her empathic openness to the emotional and spiritual effects of vicarious traumatization. These effects are cumulative and permanent, and evident in a therapist's professional and personal life." (Pearlman & Saakvitne, 1995)

Figure 2.1 (continued)

KEY CONCEPTS IN THE MATRIX OF EMPATHY

To facilitate an introduction to the concept of the matrix of empathy, we will organize and briefly identify the key concepts that constitute the psychological structure of empathy in the treatment of trauma and PTSD.

Trauma, PTSD and Related Constructs

Traumatic experiences generate a wide range of medical and psychologi-cal consequences, which include PTSD, acute stress disorders (ASD), anx-iety, mood, dissociative, substance abuse and other psychiatric disorders. Traumatization also reflects physical injuries and mental states which are not pathological in nature but may require psychotherapy (Lindy & Lifton, 2001; Wilson, Friedman, & Lindy, 2001).

Traumatic experiences may be manifest in common, universal ways across different cultures (Kinsie, 1994). Recently, the explication of the Archetype of Trauma, the Trauma Complex and Complex PTSD has been developed to characterize these universal forms of post-traumatic adap-tation (Herman, 1992; Williams & Somers, 2002; Wilson, 2002, 2003; Wilson & Drozdek, 2004; Wilson & Keane, 2004). Similarly, descriptions of the most horrifying traumatic experiences have been discussed under the rubrics of the Abyss and Inversion Experiences (Wilson, 2002, 2003; Wilson & Drozdek, 2004; Wilson & Keane, 2004) in which individuals encounter the specter of death through the demonic, pernicious, evil and dark side of human cruelty, or as determined by the capriciousness of fate. Attempts to describe the wide domain of post-traumatic phenomena have included the development of a tetrahedral model of PTSD and dissociative phenomena which contains five synergistically interacting systems of stress response patterns (Wilson, Friedman, & Lindy, 2001). These theoretical ideas expand the seminal concepts of traumatic neuro-sis, PTSD and dissociation, and point to the shifts occurring in the scientific paradigms of understanding the inner and outer world of trauma (Kalsched, 2003; Knox, 2003).

Traumatoid States

Efforts to understand the reactions and stress-related impacts of working with trauma victims have led to the development of concepts to describe the impact of this work on professional care providers, spouses, loved ones and others. Terms such as compassion fatigue (CF), borrowed stress, vicarious traumatization (VT), secondary traumatic stress (STS), second-ary traumatic stress disorder (STSD), empathic strain, empathic rupture, etc. have been developed and studied in clinical and research settings (e.g., Dalenberg, 2000; Figley, 1997, 2002; Pearlman & Saakvitne, 1995; Wilson & Lindy, 1994). In this book, we propose that a more inclusive term would be *traumatoid states* (i.e., trauma-like) as expectable reactions associated with OSRS. The concept of traumatoid states is discussed in chapters 8 and 10.

Affects, Affective States and Hyperarousal

It is a truism to say that psychological trauma produces emotional distress, pain and angst in living. The psychobiology of trauma is such that it alters the genetically wired stress response patterns in the brain and nervous system (Friedman, 2000, 2001; Friedman & McEwen, 2004; McEwen, 1998; Wilson, 2004). As part of allostatic changes in post-traumatic states, the brain and sympathetic nervous system reset baseline functioning to adapt to the stressors associated with trauma. The recalibration of the stress response system, under command and control of the neurophysiological systems in the brain, generates changes in emotional responsiveness, especially with respect to psychologically conditioned responses to stimuli and situations that have a high association value with the memory of the trauma experience. Stimuli that evoke the pre-wired stress response system may trigger affective dysregulations, resulting in intense emotional states or a recurrence of the powerful emotions connected with the original trauma experience.

As a consequence of allostatically altered psychobiological responses to trauma, the patient manifests hyperarousal states which include being "keyed up," "on edge" and "on guard"; being predisposed to overperceive threats; hypervigilance and sleep disturbance; proneness to anger and irritability; and quickness to respond in situations, especially those that evoke (consciously or unconsciously) memories of or associations with the precipitating traumatic experience.

Transference and Countertransference in Post-traumatic Therapy

The matrix of empathy plays an important role in the processes of transference and countertransference which extends beyond the classic psychoanalytic understanding of these processes. In terms of post-traumatic therapies, we will discuss several critically important aspects of transference and complex forms of countertransference:

- transmitting unconscious of traumatic states
- trauma specific transference processes (TST)
- trauma specific transference transmissions (TSTT)
- Type I and Type II countertransference reactions (CTRs)
- transference projections of traumatoid states
- encoding trauma in organismic states
- decoding trauma transmissions in seven channels
- signal detection of trauma transmission
- universal trauma themes in transference

Empathy and Related Processes

The power of trauma to alter the psychological functioning of the survivor cannot be overestimated. Depending on the nature of the traumatic experience, the impact of trauma can be subtle or overt, acute or chronic, uneventful or life altering. In the process of psychotherapy, or acting in other professional roles (e.g., physician, nurse, crisis counselor, social worker, spouse, etc.), the enactment of empathy takes many forms which require understanding and classification. A major objective of this book is to explain the dynamics of empathy in all its vicissitudes, as it influences the process of post-traumatic therapy. The conceptual complexity of empathy in the treatment of trauma and PTSD includes the following:

- qualities of empathic attunement: resonance, intensity, timing, accuracy, prediction and isochronicity
- factors determining empathic orientation: trauma history, developmental socialization, ego-maturity, life experiences and attachment capacity
- empathic identification
- empathic behavioral enactment
- empathic balance beam: balancing empathic attunement vs. empathic strain
- modes of empathic attunement: strength, accuracy, inconsistency, weakness, distancing and sufficiency
- modes of empathic strain: disequilibrium, withdrawal, enmeshment and repression
- empathic rupture and empathic breaks in professional role boundaries
- high empathic functioning
- dimensions of empathy: capacity, resistance, tolerance/sensitivity and endurance
- empathic continuum: minimal to maximal; detachment to attunement
- sustained empathic inquiry
- empathic stretch
- empathic isochronicity and the transformation of trauma

Anxiety and Defensiveness

We now have informative studies of therapists' anxiety and defensiveness in post-traumatic therapy (Dalenberg, 2000; Pearlman & Saakvitne, 1995; Thomas, 1998; Wilson & Lindy, 1994). Chapters 9 and 10 give the results of our empirical study of therapists' reactions to working with trauma clients, and the role of anxiety and defensiveness. In the context of the matrix of empathy, it is especially important to understand these processes in terms of their relationship to Type I and Type II counter-transference processes and the outcome of treatment.

ORGANIZATION OF THE BOOK

This book is constructed in such a way that the chapters are interrelated: they are conceptually and theoretically interlinked. The chapters can also be used as independent descriptions of the diverse ways in which empathy plays a role in post-traumatic therapies, no matter what the theoretical orientation (e.g., cognitive behavioral, psychodynamic, group treatment, eye movement desensitization reprocessing, pharmacological, etc.). In a holistic sense, the chapters fit together like a jigsaw puzzle. When the pieces are assembled to create the larger picture, the images become clear and are readily discerned. However, the resultant gestalt of the ideas presented resembles the perception of a piece of sculpture that changes image depending on the angle from which the free-standing structure is viewed.

Chapter 1 presents the idea initiated by Freud (1910) that unconscious processes are transmitted during treatment. In post-traumatic therapies, clients transmit information about their state of traumatization through different channels. Trauma specific transference transmission (TSTT) is one of the primary ways by which conscious and unconscious information gets transmitted from the patient (sender) to the therapist (receiver). In most cases, the data being transmitted through the seven primary channels is encoded, and reflects how the trauma experience was stored in the memory. Elements of the encoding of the trauma experience as stored, metabolized and actively processed are subsequently expressed through transference projections, symbolic manifestations, dreams, dissociative phenomena and verbal reports. We are in agreement with Freud that all actions being transmitted during treatment have meaning, as seen in the example of the combat veteran who could not remember the grizzly and horrifying details of a terrifying, night-long firefight in the jungles of Vietnam which resulted in human carnage adhering to foliage, rubber trees and blood-soaked earth. However, what was symbolic and salient was his repetitive (unconscious) action of picking at the cleats on his boots as he spoke during treatment sessions. His action had meaning and provided clues to the unmetabolized aspects of his war experiences. His unconscious continued to "pick" at the remains of friends' brains stuck in the web of his cleats.

Chapter 3 deals with the structure and dynamics of interpersonal processes in post-traumatic therapy. Here 10 structural and 10 process variables which are universal to post-traumatic therapies are identified. These dynamic processes are then placed into a conceptual overview of empathy, trauma transmission and countertransference processes in post-traumatic treatment approaches. The purpose of this conceptual model is to provide a "crow's nest" view of the universal patterns of interaction during the process of psychotherapy.

Chapter 4 gives a detailed model of empathy in trauma work. The model is then broken down into separate parts which permit magnified views of empathy in the treatment process. These magnified views are akin to looking at slides under a microscope with increasing levels of power. The mechanisms of empathy are identified as modalities of empathic attunement and empathic strain. Each of the 10 distinct modalities of empathic functioning is discussed in detail in relation to the quality of empathic functioning in psychotherapy. It is here that the concept of the *balance beam* is introduced, a term that reflects the therapist's ongoing struggle to maintain balance between modalities of empathic strain — much like a parent and child on a playground balance beam (i.e., a teeter-totter). Finally, the concept of therapeutic isochronicity is introduced in terms of the therapist's ability to sustain empathy while, at the same time, being cast into role enactments by the client (e.g., perpetrator, abusive parent, fellow combatant, internment survivor, political oppressor, judge, etc.).

Chapter 5 focuses on the problem of the balance beam and modes of empathic attunement/strain. The chapter begins by defining the functional and process dimensions associated with qualities of empathy (i.e., resonance, intensity, accuracy, prediction, isochronicity and timing). Similarly, the core dimensions of empathy which underlie the qualities of empathic attunement are discussed. These core dimensions include empathic capacity, empathic resistance, empathic tolerance/sensitivity and empathic endurance. Based on the dynamic interrelationship between the core dimensions of empathy and the qualities of empathic attunement, it is possible to derive detailed descriptions of the personality and behavioral characteristics of persons with high versus low empathic ability. This is especially useful since identification of the high empathy therapist specifies behavioral dimensions which can be studied systematically in relation to treatment outcomes.

Chapter 6 discusses the rupture of empathy and the concept of affect dysregulation in the therapist. Building on the seminal work of Wilson and Lindy (1994), the discussion expands the analysis of Type I and Type II CTRs and their operation during the course of treatment. The dynamics of the rupture in empathy and resultant pathogenic consequences to treatment is also discussed, illustrating, through a case example, how the rupture of empathy and loss of therapeutic role boundaries can lead to any or all of the following outcomes: (1) cessation or termination in the recovery process; (2) fixation within a phase of recovery; (3) regression in the service of the ego and personal security; (4) intensification of transference issues; (5) acting out; and (6) dissociative processes. The chapter concludes with an analysis of 10 universal themes of TST and behavioral dispositions in post-traumatic therapy.

Chapter 7 covers anxiety and defensiveness in the therapist during the course of post-traumatic therapy. Recent research has identified a set of symptoms, reactions and behaviors which signify the presence of persistent tension, anxiety and defensiveness in the therapist as evoked by the client. The chapter examines the personality traits of therapists and how they are related to modes of empathic attunement, modes of empathic strain and Type I or Type II countertransference processes. Next, a review of several studies of anxiety, defensiveness and countertransference is presented, highlighting the common themes, reactions, symptoms and problems encountered by therapists who work with victims of trauma. The importance of affect dysregulation in the therapist as the counterpart to affect dysregulation in clients with PTSD and comorbidities is emphasized. The discussion concludes with a summary model of affect dysregulation, anxiety states, coping and defense in post-traumatic therapies.

Chapter 8 analyzes empathy in relation to the concept of traumatoid states. The purpose of this chapter is to examine the effects of exposure to trauma clients on the helping professional. The analysis highlights the differences between compassion fatigue (CF), vicarious traumatization (VT) and secondary traumatic stress disorder (STSD). These three concepts have been developed to explain the formation of stress-related symptoms, reactions and behaviors that have similarity to PTSD symptoms. However, a careful study of the definitions of these concepts (Figley, 2000; Pearlman & Saakvitne, 1995) would show that they all emanate through the process of empathic identification with the client. It is suggested that empathic identification leads to empathic strain, involving states of affect dysregulation in the professional therapist. Therefore, with repeated exposure to traumatized clients, the stress-evoked states in the helping professional may be associated with the transformation of self-capacities, that is, vicarious traumatization, feelings of compassion fatigue (i.e., mental fatigue and costs of caring) and secondary traumatic stress reaction (i.e., traumatoid states akin to PTSD symptoms).

By differentiating between the types of stress-evoked response patterns reported by mental health professionals working with trauma clients, it becomes possible to define more precisely the nature of these OSRS as traumatoid states, or those that are "trauma-like" but, in fact, are fundamentally different, since the helping professional's involvement with trauma clients does not usually involve direct exposure to a life-threatening or traumatic event that would meet the prime diagnostic criteria for PTSD (A_1, A_2). However, as discussed in chapter 10, the concept of traumatoid states is operationalizable, and can be meaningfully defined in precise terms which include the concepts of CF, VT and STSD. Further, the concept of traumatoid states has 10 separate dimensions: (1) dysregulated affective states; (2) empathic identification; (3) empathic strain; (4) somatic symptoms (e.g., headaches, fatigue, sleep disturbance); (5) altered self-capacities; (6) personal and professional CTRs; (7) difficulties in disclosing the stress-related effects of the work; (8) altered stress thresholds; (9) allo-static manifestations of stress response; and (10) altered conceptualization of spirituality. These 10 dimensions of traumatoid states enable the possi-bility of creating a new diagnostic category for OSRS, using the same log-ical and algorithmic criteria as contained in the diagnostic and statistical manual of the American Psychiatric Association (*Diagnostic and Statistical Manual-IV-TR*, 2000).

Chapters 9 and 10 report on the results of a large-scale study of profes-sional mental health workers who work with trauma clients and PTSD. In chapter 9, results of the study utilizing the Clinicians' Trauma Reaction Survey (CTRS; Thomas & Wilson, 1996) are reported. Using a factor analytic statistical procedure, the CTRS was analyzed and produced five distinct factor structures: (1) intrusive preoccupation with trauma; (2) avoidance and detachment; (3) overinvolvement and identification; (4) professional alienation; and (5) professional role satisfaction. The results of this study provide strong empirical support for the existence of empathic strains and Type I and Type II countertransference patterns described by Wilson and Lindy (1994). The Appendix gives the CTRS.

In Chapter 10, the results of the CTRS are examined in great detail, the purpose being to explore the nature and validity of traumatoid states, vicarious traumatization, compassion fatigue and the modalities of empathic attunement and empathic strain. The chapter systematically addresses and answers critical questions which include the following: Does work with trauma clients meet the A_1 and A_2 diagnostic criteria for PTSD? Are symptoms of PTSD present among helping professionals who are repeatedly exposed to trauma clients as a result of the work itself? What effects, if any, does trauma work have on the identity of the helping professional? Does work with trauma victims impact the professional's worldview, sense of meaning, beliefs and ideology? Are the stress-evoked effects of doing professional trauma work expressed in dysregulated affective states and somatic symptoms? Do professionals who work with trauma victims have difficulty in maintaining professional role bound-aries and in disclosing the nature of their CTRs? What evidence is there for the existence of a unique stress response syndrome, characterized as a traumatoid state, as a result of the work? Trauma therapists and trauma clients — who chooses whom? This question is examined, and empirical data reveal complex and fascinating questions and answers about the nature of post-traumatic therapy itself.

Chapter 11 highlights the positive therapeutic effects of empathic attune-ment. The discussion returns to the fundamental question of how trauma evokes (negative) allostatic changes in prolonged stress response syndromes. PTSD, in particular, is a manifestation of a dysregulated stress response system which is psychobiological in nature (Friedman, 2000, 2001). By understanding how traumatic experiences evoke negative allostasis, the question can then be asked as to how they get transformed into positive allostatic states. How do traumatized states get transformed into healthy ones? We suggest that empathic attunement is the key to the transformation of negative allostatic states into positive allostatic ones. This transformation is a resetting and recalibration of organismic functioning which is identified as the process of organismic tuning. More specifically, the processes of empathic attunement, isochronicity and dyschronicity in the course of treatment are presented and related to overmodulated, undermodulated and variably modulated states in the therapist during the course of post-traumatic therapy. Next, the discussion clarifies that, with sustained empathic attunement, 15 distinct aspects of positive allostasis are discernible. These 15 dimensions reflect positive transformation in states of traumatization which are associated with psychological health and optimal states of functioning.

REFERENCES

American Psychiatric Association. (2000). *Diagnostic and statistical manual of mental disorders* (4th ed., text rev.). Washington, DC: Author.

Aronoff, J. & Wilson, J. P. (1985). *Personality in the social process*. Livingston, NJ: Erlbaum.

Dalenberg, C. (2000). *Countertransference and PTSD*. Washington, DC: American Psychological Association Press.

Dalenberg, C. L. (2000). *Countertransference in the treatment of trauma*. Washington, DC: American Psychological Association Press.

Eisenberg, N., Murphy, B. C. & Shepard, S. (1997). Developmental aspects of empathic accuracy. In W. Ickes (Ed.), *Empathic accuracy* (pp. 73–117). New York: Guilford Publications.

Figley, C. (1995). *Compassion fatigue*. New York: Brunner/Mazel.

Figley, C. (2002). *Treating compassion fatigue*. New York: Brunner-Routledge.

Friedman, M. J. (2000). *Posttraumatic and acute stress disorders*. Kansas City, MO: Compact Clinicals.

Friedman, M. J. (2000). *Post-traumatic stress disorder: The latest assessment and treatment strategies*. Kansas City, MO: Compact Clinicals.

Friedman, M. J. (2001). Allostatic versus empirical perspectives on pharmacotherapy. In J. P. Wilson, M. J. Friedman, & J. D. Lindy (Eds.), *Treating psychological trauma and PTSD* (pp. 94–125). New York: Guilford Publications.

Friedman, M. (in press). Psychobiology and pharmacological approaches to treatment. In *The international handbook of traumatic stress syndromes*. New York: Plenum Press.

Friedman, M. J. & McEwen, B. S. (2004). PTSD, allostatic load and medical illness. In P. P. Schnurr & B. L. Green (Eds.), *Trauma and health: Physical consequences of exposure to extreme stress* (pp. 157–189). Washington, DC: American Psychological Association.

Herman, J. (1992). *Trauma and recovery*. New York: Basic Books.

Kalsched, D. (2003). Daimonic elements in early trauma. *Journal of Analytical Psychology, 48*(2), 145–176.

Kinsie, J. D. (1994). Countertransference in the treatment of Southeast Asian refugees. In J. P. Wilson & J. D. Lindy (Eds.), *Countertransference in the treatment of PTSD* (pp. 245–249). New York: Guilford Publications.

Knox, J. (2003). Trauma and defenses: Their roots in relationship: An overview. *Journal of Analytical Psychology, 48,* 207–233.

Kohut, H. (1971). *The analysis of the self.* New York: International Universities Press.

Lindy, J. D. & Lifton, R. J. (2001). *Beyond invisible walls.* New York: Brunner-Routledge.

McEwen, B. (1998). Protective and damaging effects of stress mediators. *Seminars of the Beth Israel Deaconess Medical Center, 338*(3), 171–179.

Pearlman, L. & Saakvitne, K. (1995). *Trauma and the therapist.* New York: Norton.

Staub, E. (1979). *Positive social behavior and morality.* New York: Academic Press.

Thomas, R. B. (1998). *An investigation of empathic stress reactions among mental health professionals working with PTSD.* Unpublished doctoral dissertation, Union Institute, Cincinnati, OH.

Thomas, R. B. & Wilson, J. P. (1996). *Clinicians' trauma reaction survey (CTRS).* Cleveland, OH: John P. Wilson, Cleveland State University.

Williams, M. B. & Somers, J. (2002). *Simple and complex PTSD.* New York: Haworth Press.

Wilson, J. P. (2002, October). *The abyss experience and catastrophic stress.* Presentation at St. Joseph's University, Terrorism and Weapons of Mass Destruction, Philadelphia, PA.

Wilson, J. P. (2003, February). *Target goals and interventions for PTSD: From trauma to the abyss experience.* Paper presented at the meeting of the International Critical Incident Stress Foundation, 7th World Congress on Stress, Trauma and Coping, Baltimore, MD.

Wilson, J. P. (2004). Broken spirits. In J. P. Wilson & B. Drozdek (Eds.), *Broken spirits: The treatment of traumatized asylum seekers, refugees and war and torture victims* (pp. 141–173). New York: Brunner-Routledge.

Wilson, J. P. & Drozdek, B. (2004). *Broken spirits: The treatment of traumatized asylum seekers, refugees and war and torture victims.* New York: Brunner-Routledge.

Wilson, J. P., Friedman, M. J. & Lindy, J. D. (2001). *Treating psychological trauma and PTSD.* New York: Guilford Publications.

Wilson, J. P. & Keane, T. M. (2004). *Assessing psychological trauma and PTSD* (2nd ed.). New York: Guilford Publications.

Wilson, J. & Lindy, J. (1994). *Countertransference in the treatment of PTSD.* New York: Guilford Publications.

3

Structure and Dynamics of Interpersonal Processes in Treatment of PTSD

The course of treatment of trauma patients is a journey, like the myth of the Hero described so brilliantly by Joseph Campbell (1949) in his book *Hero with a Thousand Faces*. In the universal myth of the Hero, an ordinary individual encounters, at some point in his life journey, profoundly frightening and traumatic difficulties — life-changing experiences such as involvement in warfare, life-threatening illness, a battle with severe mental illness or addiction, sudden loss of family or one's culture, and devastating effects of catastrophe, such as the terrorist attacks on the World Trade Center in 2001. In the story of the Hero, the protagonist encounters powerful forces of a dangerous and foreboding nature. These strong forces constitute a zone of danger to the soul, spirit, identity and life itself. As the journey proceeds, a guardian spirit, nurturant elder or God may assist in the task of persevering through the treacherous zone of danger and the encounter with supernatural forces. It is an upward struggle out of darkness, despair and the abyss where soul and identity are tested. After enduring peril, turmoil and the specter of death, the Hero emerges with a new perspective of himself, with unrealized strength, potential and power which await unification in an emergent self.

Clinical work with trauma and PTSD is very much like the journey of Joseph Campbell's mythical Hero, who has "thousands of faces" in the history of humankind and the mythology of anthropology. The therapist who chooses to work with traumatized persons will encounter the many faces of physical and psychological trauma. The faces and voices of their stories vary, but their spiritual journey is the same: to overcome the darkness of their trauma experiences and regain wholeness of personality.

There is nothing easy in the journey for either the doctor/therapist/ helper or the patient/client/victim. To make the journey requires that trauma survivors revisit the experiences that altered their sense of themselves as persons. In complementary fashion, the therapist must be able to accompany the patient as a guide on pathways of recovery and psychic integration. The psychotherapy of patients with PTSD is demanding and fraught with risks and difficulties for the guide acting in the role of the therapist. These guides, like the Hero, will confront the darkness of being and unimagined forces which will test the limits of their professional training. These risks and difficulties have been documented in recent research, and include the development of empathic distress in the therapist by exposure to the trauma narratives of clients (Dalenberg, 2000; Figley, 2002; Wilson & Drozdek, 2004).

Empathic attunement is a vehicle of entry into the trauma client's inner world. Immersion into this inner world of traumatization can be fear provoking, overwhelmingly distressful, and anxiety producing and can lead to altered views on humanity, morality, justice and the goodness of life (Pearlman & Saakvitne, 1995). Such immersion through empathic attunement also means immersion into the ego-space of traumatized persons and the realm of the abyss—the intense emotional cauldron of dysregulated affective states and their expression in altered patterns of attachment relationships. Indeed, it is the nature of traumatic experiences to create extremely complex states of psychic traumatization. The therapist, in a professional helping role, seeks to understand the nature of traumatization, and will inevitably be "pulled in" by the sheer power of the trauma transference (Dalenberg, 2000). Listening empathically to the trauma narrative and its impact on the altered quality of a patient's life may cause the therapist to become absorbed in trauma material, like entering a zone of virtual reality in three-dimensional space. As the therapist gets pulled into the patient's inner world of traumatization and the magnetic force of his or her trauma story and personal state of injury, the stark reality and devastating extent of the patient's trauma experience may become so real that it seems like the therapist's own experience. Realities and boundaries may blur, creating states of confusion. This phenomenon has been variously labeled vicarious traumatization, secondary traumatization, empathic distress, compassion fatigue, trauma-related countertransference, and affective overloading (Figley, 2002, 1995; Wilson & Lindy, 1994).

In describing the nature of vicarious traumatization, Pearlman and Saakvitne (1995) state,

> vicarious traumatization refers to a *transformation in the therapist's* (or other trauma worker's) *inner experience* resulting from empathic engagement with the client's trauma material. That is, through exposure to clients' graphic accounts of sexual abuse experiences and to the realities of people's intentional cruelty to one another, and through the inevitable re-enactments in the therapy relationship, the therapist is vulnerable through his or her *empathic openness* to the emotional and spiritual effects of vicarious

traumatization. These effects are *cumulative and permanent*, and evident in a therapist's professional and personal life. (p. 151, italics ours)

Pearlman and Saakvitne (1995) state,

One of our most valued tools is our capacity to enter *empathically* into the experience of our clients. The therapist's *empathy is essential* to the creation of a therapeutic relationship and thus recovery ... *yet empathy also puts us at risk for vicarious traumatization*; in particular, *a specific type of empathic connection* with our clients can heighten vicarious traumatization. (p. 296, italics ours)

These clinical insights are informative, because they highlight the fact that the treatment of trauma and PTSD is a dual unfolding process with its own structure and dynamics (Wilson & Lindy, 1994). Moreover, while the exercise of empathy in the course of post-traumatic therapies is critical, it can also be viewed as a double-edged sword which cuts both ways. The dual unfolding process reflects the fact that, in the treatment dyad (or group context), the journey of discovery during the treatment process is one that unfolds for both participants as the interpersonal dynamics get played out. The traumatized patient relives, reenacts and reexperiences all aspects of the trauma experience at multiple levels of psychological functioning: dysregulated affect; cognitive information processing (including traumatic memory encoding); perceptual processes; and altered response tendencies and behavioral dispositions. Clearly, these are organismically based changes induced by trauma and involve allostatic disruptions, reflecting prolonged stress response and adaptive behaviors (McEwen, 1998; Wilson, Friedman, & Lindy, 2001).

On the other side of the coin in the dual unfolding process, the therapist, through the vehicle of empathic attunement, experiences the disastrous impact on the client and the client's state of traumatization. This impact has been labeled trauma specific transference (TST) by Wilson and Lindy (1994), meaning that transference reenactments, and transference projections of the patient's ego and organismic states, get transferred dynamically in the therapeutic relationship to the therapist. This set of dynamic transference processes, in essence, recapitulates the traumatic mechanisms which disturbed intrapsychic processes at the time of the traumatic event(s). The nature of this psychic disturbance impacts the existing self-structure and ego-identity of the client (Wilson, 2004). The traumatic transferences, in all of their vicissitudes, interweave major aspects of the therapeutic relationship: affective attachments; self-object (therapist) relations; affective processing; intimacy bonding; evolved role differentiation in dyadic style; evoked feelings of love and sexuality (Coen, 2002); and the understanding of meaning by the patient and therapist of how the shared trauma experience affected their lives. For the therapist, this set of impacts on the therapeutic process extends to both professional and personal life (see chapter 10 for a discussion). In this sense, we can return to our metaphoric image of Joseph Campbell's mythical Hero, who encounters the forces of overwhelming power and darkness, struggles with deep, soul-searching uncertainty, and then emerges with the capacity for self-transfiguration. So, too, the dual unfolding process of post-traumatic treatments for trauma and PTSD carries the participants on a shared journey of the unknown.

STRUCTURE, PROCESS AND DYNAMICS IN THE TREATMENT OF PTSD

Empathy is a multidimensional construct whose dimensions include intellectual skills; cognitive abilities to conceptualize the internal working models of the patient's state of traumatization; the capacity for accurately recognizing and communicating understanding of emotions, thought processes and nonverbal messages through different body channels (e.g., face, voice, posture, movement, etc.); and the capacity to modulate one's own affective reactions in order to maintain resonance and attunement. Conceptually, empathy can be construed as a psychological state with varying properties similar to different forms of love, affection and sorrow (Coen, 2003). The varying degrees of empathy and empathic skills can facilitate or hinder progress during treatment, that is, create a relational climate that assists the traumatized patient in working through the impact of trauma on the individual sense of well-being.

To fully appreciate the central role of empathy in the treatment of trauma patients, it is useful and necessary to delineate the structure and process of treatment in a general way. In an overly simplified sense, structure refers to the identifiable organizational framework and interrelated components that comprise post-traumatic therapies (see Wilson, Friedman, & Lindy, 2001, for a review). For example, some treatment approaches for PTSD are highly structured, such as cognitive behavioral therapies (CBT) and eye movement desensitization reprocessing (EMDR). Other treatments are less structured (e.g., psychoanalysis) and evolve over time, as issues of treatment emerge during the process. Still other treatments (e.g., pharmacotherapy) focus narrowly on symptom reduction through the use of medication. Indeed, if patients undergoing comparably different types of post-traumatic treatment were videotaped, observers would be able to identify structural differences: eye movements in EMDR; anxiety reduction desensitization procedures in CBT; free association and dream reports in analytical approaches; statements of symptom reduction in pharmacotherapy; increased interpersonal activity and personal confrontations in group treatment approaches. However, no

I.	Inception of Treatment: time frame and contract
II.	Context of Treatment: setting (e.g., clinic, hospital, private)
III.	Role Differentiation: hierarchical vs. egalitarian in professional-clinical relationship
IV	Length of Treatment, Treatment Objective, Criterion of Outcome
V.	Emergent Trauma Related Themes and Issues
VI.	Symptom Presentation, Subjective Distress, Adaptive Functionality of Client
VII.	Traumatic Transference Reactions
VIII.	Explicit or Implicit Boundaries in Role Differentiation
IX.	Supervisory and Consultation Mechanisms
X.	Termination of Treatment Processes

Figure 3.1 Structural dimensions of post-traumatic therapies (PTT). Copyright John P. Wilson, 2003.

matter which treatment approach is applied, a videotaped chronological record would indicate the presence of discernible structural dimensions which are listed below and summarized in Figure 3.1.

STRUCTURAL DIMENSIONS IN POST-TRAUMATIC THERAPIES

- Inception of treatment (time frame)
- Context of treatment setting (hospital, office, group, etc.)
- Role differentiation (e.g., professional vs. client)
- Length of time and number of sessions (duration)
- Emergent trauma-related themes (e.g., intrusive violation, catastrophic disaster, witnessing horror, political oppression, abandonment, humiliation, loss, etc.)
- Symptom presentations and reports (e.g., PTSD, anxiety, self-pathologies)
- Traumatic transference reactions (TST, TSTT)
- Explicit or implicit boundaries in role differentiation (limits, rules)
- Supervisory regulation (e.g., self-disclosure, countertransference)
- Termination and end of treatment (conclusion)

These 10 structural dimensions can be analyzed across different treatment modalities, at any given time, to provide a comparative and cross-sectional picture of how the traumatized client is holding out in terms of working through the traumatic experience. Horowitz and colleagues (Horowitz, 1976, 1986, 1993) used such an approach in time-limited treatment (12–16 weeks), in which different aspects of post-traumatic recovery formed the target objectives of treatment at specified time intervals (beginning, middle and end phases). Zoellner, Fitzgibbons, & Foa

(2001) have detailed cognitive behavioral treatments within time-limited frameworks. Similarly, Lindy (1993) has described focal psychoanalytic approaches to PTSD treatment by delineating key themes which emerge during the initial, middle and end phases of psychodynamic uncovering techniques without a specified time limit. Foy et al. (2001) have reviewed the efficacy of time-limited group treatment (12–16 weeks) for combat veterans and noted their relative effectiveness in reducing chronic PTSD symptoms. Thus, every therapeutic approach contains an *underlying structure* which governs the process of dyadic or group interaction. Moreover, despite differences in approaches to treating traumatized patients with different types of trauma experiences, the therapist will inevitably experience professional and personal reactions during the process which also have discernible dimensions. Figure 3.2 summarizes these dimensions.

PROCESS DIMENSIONS IN POST-TRAUMATIC THERAPIES

- Affective reactions (dysregulated affective states, empathic strains, compassion fatigue, vicarious traumatization)
- Boundary regulations and management
- Therapeutic alliance maintenance
- Empathic process: modalities of empathic attunement vs. empathic strain
- Therapeutic skills and clinical techniques
- Assessments of treatment progress
- Cognition and perceptions of patient's symptoms in relation to formulation of treatment plan and target objectives
- Determination of treatment efficacy/outcomes

I.	Affective Reactions, Dysregulation and Manifestations
II.	Boundary Regulations and Management
III.	Countertransference Regulation and Management
IV.	Therapeutic Alliance, Trust, Safety and Stability
V.	Empathic Process: Attunement vs. Strain
VI.	Level of Clinical and Therapeutic Scales
VII.	Assessment of Treatment Progress
VIII.	Cognition and Formulations of Client's Trauma Related Symptoms
IX.	Formulations of Treatment Plan and Target Objectives
X.	Criteria and Determination of Treatment Efficacy and Outcomes

Figure 3.2 Process dimensions of post-traumatic therapies (PTT). Copyright John P. Wilson, 2003.

From a dynamic interactional perspective of post-traumatic therapy, 10 *process variables* are linked with structural dimensions in the treatment setting. Likewise, a videotaped chronology of the process of treatment would permit analysis of these dimensions as well. To cite a few examples: What was the therapist's affective reaction to a patient's account of rape, torture, sexual abuse, loss of body parts or witnessing massive death scenes? How was a boundary issue dealt with if a patient expresses hate, love, self-loathing or a desire for sex with the therapist (Coen, 2003)? What if the therapist's competence and credibility is directly challenged? What if the patient does not improve, despite clinical efforts, consultation and supervision? What if the intensity of treatment sessions is so great that the therapist experiences chronic doubt, anxiety, uncertainty and affective dysregulation (i.e., severe prolonged empathic strain)? And, what if the reports of the trauma patient's experience challenge long-standing personal beliefs about morality, religion, faith, and core beliefs about human nature and the goodness of life?

It is apparent that the issues of therapeutic structure and dynamic processes are linked in extremely complex and interactive ways. The processes of empathy are like a gyroscope in navigating the course of treatment. In this regard, it is critical to understand the mechanisms that sustain empathic attunement, and the forces that contribute to empathic strain, compassion fatigue, vicarious traumatization and countertransference processes in post-traumatic modalities of treatment, crisis debriefing and other forms of professional trauma work.

A CONCEPTUAL SCHEMA OF STRUCTURAL AND PROCESS DIMENSIONS IN POST-TRAUMATIC TREATMENT APPROACHES

Figure 3.3 presents a conceptual schema of structural and process dimensions in post-traumatic treatment approaches. This conceptual schema illustrates the "flow" of dual unfolding processes in treatment. Following Racker's (1968) observation that transference and countertransference are indigenous to psychodynamic treatment, we can see that forms of TST and their related counterparts in countertransference unfold in the therapeutic dyad over time. Hence, the term *dual unfolding* is not only descriptive of a process but it also points to the jointly placed journey of discovery that ensues between therapist and patient.

Allan Schore (2003a, 2003b) has written three comprehensive volumes on affective dysregulation with special application to PTSD. As a prolonged stress response which becomes disordered, PTSD has, as one of its hallmark features, the omnipresence of *dysregulated affects* which emanate from the trauma experience. As part of allostatic changes in how the brain adapts to prolonged stress states, the PTSD patient often presents with intense affect when reliving, reexperiencing or recounting

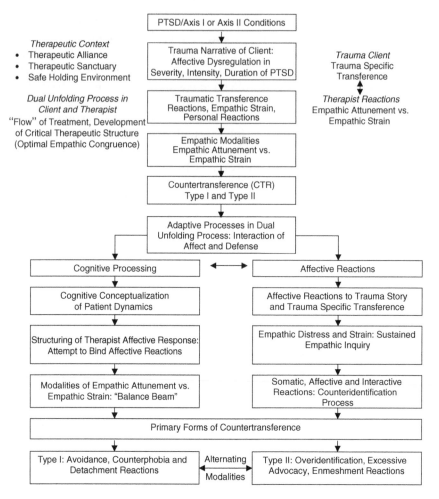

Figure 3.3 Empathy and countertransference in post-traumatic therapies. Copyright John P. Wilson, 2003; John P. Wilson and Jacob D. Lindy, 1994.

memories of the trauma experience. However, depending on the nature and control functions of ego-defenses, they may appear emotionally flat, constricted and psychically numb to the trauma events. Thus, the telling of the trauma story (narrative) will vary over time in terms of the severity, frequency and intensity of affective dysregulation. Schore (2003a) has discussed the nature of dysregulation of the right brain hemisphere in PTSD:

The emotional disturbances of PTSD have been suggested to have their origins in the inability of the right prefrontal cortex to *modulate* amygdala functions ... Morgan and LeDoux (1995) conclude that without orbital prefrontal feedback regarding the level of threat, the organism remains in an amygdala—driven *defensive response* state longer than necessary, that in humans, conditioned fear acquisition and extinction are associated with right hemispheres dominant amygdala function (LeBar et al., 1998) and that a defective orbitofrontal system operates in PTSD (Moyer et al. (1993). (p. 239, italics ours)

Moreover, as part of this complex neurological system governing adaptation to traumatic stressors, the dysregulation in the right hemisphere of the brain activates mechanisms that make pathological dissociative states an integral part of adaptive and protective organismic responses to trauma. Schore (2003a, 2003b) describes this process:

The neuroscience literature also indicates that *dissociation* is associated with a deficiency in the right brain. Crucian and colleagues described a dissociation between the *emotional evaluation* of an event and the physiological reaction to that event, with the process being intact on right hemisphere function. ... A failure of orbitofrontal function is seen in the hypometabolic state of *pathological dissociation*, and this dysfunction would interfere with its normal role in processing motivational information and *modulating* the motivational control of goal-directed behavior, and therefore manifest as a deficit in organizing the expression of a regulated emotional response and an appropriate motivational state for a particular social environmental context. (p. 137, italics ours)

The PTSD patient presents in treatment with a *preset* psychobiological disposition to manifest varying degrees of affect dysregulation as a kind of infrastructure to the full-blown cluster of PTSD symptoms which include changes in the self-structure and fluctuating ego-states (e.g., hypervigilance, rage, fear, helplessness, dissociation, hyperarousal, etc.). Since psychotherapy has a circumscribed therapeutic context, the patient's initial perceptions of the therapist's capacity to be genuinely empathic, understanding and capable of "holding" (i.e., sustained empathic empathy) are important, and will influence the pattern of trauma related transferences which, of course, will likewise "unfold" and change in their dynamics over time. Therefore, the combination of strong affect dysregulation, proneness to dissociation and testing the therapist's capacity to "receive" the trauma story always exists as treatment begins. As noted by many clinicians (Chu, 1999; Courtois, 1999; Parson, 1988; Pearlman & Saakvitne, 1995), the creation of a safe therapeutic sanctuary is essential to facilitate the "flow" and disclosure of information on how the patient's sense of well-being was compromised by her or his traumatization. Further, with good initial empathic attunement, a *critical therapeutic structure* develops which will undergo transformations in the dynamics of the dual unfolding process between the patient and the therapist. As the therapy progresses, the patient will disclose more and more trauma related affects, sharpen the depth and clarity of the memories of aspects of the trauma and seek to process the experiences in ways that are more congruent with self-schematas (Horowitz, 1986). At the same time, as a reciprocal part of the dual unfolding process, the therapist will experience empathic strains, distressing and dysregulated affect states and her or his own reactions to the trauma story. In a parallel way, the therapist seeks to understand the patient's trauma experience through personal empathic reactions and cognitive processing attempts to interpret, as accurately as possible, what was presented and/or projected by trauma specific transferences.

EMPATHIC MODALITIES: EMPATHIC ATTUNEMENT VS. EMPATHIC STRAINS

As illustrated in Figure 3.3, the two principal modalities of empathy are central to understanding the nature and dynamics of the dual unfolding process. We have listed six modalities of empathic attunement and four modalities of empathic strain to describe qualities of the communication patterns and styles of interaction in the therapeutic dyad. In chapter 5, these dimensions are explored in greater detail under the rubric of the balance beam which reflects the processes by which empathic attunement and empathic strain counterbalance each other. Ideally, of course, the therapist attempts to sustain good empathic attunement. However, the power of the client's trauma stories may be so great that this is not possible. When significant empathic strain occurs, the balance beam tilts towards the side of one of the modes of empathic strain (i.e., withdrawal, repression, disequilibrium, enmeshment) and leads to momentary shifts away from empathic attunement. As discussed in chapter 6, accurate, recurrent or unexpected empathic strain may lead to either Type I (avoidant, counterphobic, detachment) or Type II (overidentification, excessive advocacy, enmeshment) CTRs. Type I and Type II CTRs may, in turn, cause ruptures in the fabric of empathy in the relationship, potentially damaging the flow and progression of post-traumatic recovery. However, the presence of empathic strains in themselves can significantly effect adaptive processes in the dual unfolding process. Specifically, this refers to the interaction of affects (especially dysregulated affects) and defenses in the therapist.

ADAPTIVE PROCESSES IN DUAL UNFOLDING PROCESSES: AFFECT AND DEFENSE

For purposes of illustration, Figure 3.3 divides the naturally occurring cognitive and affective processes into separate components to show the interactive nature of these processes which are themselves integrally linked to empathic modalities.

First, whether there is good empathic attunement or empathic strain, the therapist formulates his or her own understanding of the patient's reports, history, trauma narrative and associative mental processes during the treatment sessions. This is a process of cognitive conceptualization of the patient's dynamics and is, of course, influenced by many factors which include character, training and clinical experience. At the same time, the therapist experiences *affective reactions* while listening to the trauma story, reacting to states of affect dysregulation in the patient, and attempting to process TST behaviors. In terms of dyadic flow, the therapists aim to structure their personal emotional reactions—to bind anxiety, doubt, sadness, uncertainty or other affects in an attempt to sustain empathic attunement. This process may occur outside of conscious awareness and simultaneously generate *somatic reactions* (e.g., headache, muscle tension, stomach upset, urinary urgency, etc.) and *associative thoughts* (e.g., fantasies of escape, thoughts about personal outside activities, resentment towards the client, etc.).

The presence in the therapist of *unmodulated affective arousal*, associated with one of the four primary modalities of empathic strain, may lead to (1) rupture of empathic attunement; (2) Type I or Type II CTR; (3) rekindling of memories of the therapist's personal trauma, emotional abuse or neglect or, more generally, strong feelings of vulnerability and professional uncertainty as to the correct clinical procedures to follow. This phenomenon has been described poignantly by M. J. Tansey and W. F. Burke (1989) in their book, *Understanding Countertransference*:

> Defensive activity is then set in motion unconsciously in the therapist, *blocking from consciousness the potential signal value of the affective impact* of the identificatory experience. This defensive posture, for example, may surface in the therapist becoming "too nice" in an attempt to compensate for unconscious guilt, anger, or sadistic impulses towards a patient. On the other hand, a therapist who feels gratified by a patient's idealization may block his pleasure from awareness by an excessively stiff or formal approach. In the therapist, the unfortunate outcome of his defensive activity is a *countertransference impact without the absolutely vital awareness that this impact has occurred*. Although a projective identification *transmitted* by the patient has taken hold within, the therapist cannot move forward in the internal processing phase without becoming more aware that this critical event has in fact taken place. The *empathic process may simply arrest at this point*. If the disruption is *severe, regression in the empathic process* may also occur in which the therapist reacts to unconscious identificatory experience by abruptly revisiting, in one form or another, further interactional pressure without even becoming aware of the underlying emotions that have been blocked from consciousness. A regression from this level may

also disturb and disrupt a therapist's heretofore intact mental state. (p. 82, italics ours)

This quote from Tansey and Burke's (1989) clinical research clearly highlights the significance and relationship of empathy to potential countertransference processes, either Type I ("an excessively stiff or formal response") or Type II ("becoming too nice in an attempt to compensate for unconscious guilt, anger, or sadistic impulses"). Moreover, since empathy is a primary vehicle for obtaining knowledge of the patient's internal working models of the trauma experience, the disruption in the quality of modes of empathic attunement, by the interactive "here and now" operation of affects and defenses utilized to modulate them, may cause the empathic process to "simply arrest." As Figure 3.3 shows, the impact of the patient's transferences will not cease, even if "empathy arrests" at some point in time because of an empathic strain and the interaction of affects and defenses. Nevertheless, the internal cognitive processing of information does not terminate (cf. "defensive activity is then set in motion unconsciously … blocking from consciousness the potential signal value of the affective impact of the identificatory experience"). The balance between modalities of empathic attunement and empathic strain becomes critically important for maintaining what Freud (1917) described as "evenly hovering attention" in order to accurately track the stream of the patient's actions during the course of treatment.

DEVELOPMENT OF AN OPTIMAL AND CRITICAL THERAPEUTIC STRUCTURE

As illustrated in Figure 3.3, the development of an optimal therapeutic structure is essential for the successful treatment of trauma patients and PTSD. Wilson and Lindy (1994) define a *critical therapeutic structure* (CTS) as

a safe holding environment with clear and appropriate role boundaries, in which the *survivor's affects* and *therapist's empathic strain* are successfully managed. (p. 34, italics ours)

To achieve an optimal therapeutic structure, it is imperative for the trauma therapist to remain open, and to acknowledge and discuss, through supervision/consultation, the nature of the empathic strains, states of affective distress (e.g., confusion, anger, sorrow) and different forms of CTR (cf. objective, indigenous normative reactions vs. personal, subjective idiosyncratic reactions). An optimal and critical therapeutic structure enables the construction of a milieu of safety, trust, security and protection in the therapist's office—a safe sanctuary—where the patient feels that emotional burdens can be understood, lessened in weight and "contained" by a genuinely caring therapist. The perception of having an inviolate, safe sanctuary facilitates the patient's being open and "unloading" the most burdensome aspects of the trauma experiences. Transference processes will naturally occur in such environments, and several authors (e.g., Dalenberg, 2000; Herman, 1992; Pearlman & Saatvikne, 1995) have remarked on the sheer intensity of both transference and countertransference processes in work with traumatized patients. Since traumatic events are among the most extreme forms of human experience, often dealing with issues of life and death, it is to be expected that the post-traumatic emotional sequelae will carry over into treatment, much like the outer edge of shock waves from an atomic bomb explosion, or the residual winds as rains from a hurricane blow ashore and move inland.

TRAUMA SPECIFIC TRANSFERENCE AND EMPATHIC STRETCH

In post-traumatic therapies, the therapist is the recipient of the tidal-wave effects of trauma. The "gale-force" winds jolt the solemnity of the therapist's clinic, causing powerful impacts on the therapist's stability and capacity to remain professionally anchored amid such turbulent pressures. Trauma specific transference (TST) contains within itself the embeddedness of the patient's trauma experiences. The embeddedness of psychic trauma ranges from the surface level to deep inner layers which may be carefully hidden.

Wilson and Lindy (1994, p. 58) have identified five components of TST: (1) the imagery content of the trauma story; (2) the complexity and intensity of the trauma experience; (3) the clarity or ambiguity of transference projections and their accurate perception and resolution by the therapist; (4) the nature and dynamics of trauma transference themes; and (5) the affect arousal potential (AAP) of TST for the therapist. As Figure 3.3 shows, these five dimensions of TST reactions strongly affect the empathic modalities at work during the course of treatment.

Exposure to a "Big Bang" trauma story inevitably produces strong personal reactions in the listener, similar to the impact of the original event on the trauma client. Stories of extreme cruelty, which defy the moral decency of basic humanity and human rights, immediately strike resonant discord and engender disbelief, disavowal and denial, or inflame anger and desires for retribution and justice. For example, here is a case history on which I (JPW) was asked to consult, while working in Bosnia during the war years (1993–1995). It is the case of a female Bosnian Muslim survivor of ethnic cleansing during the Balkan war in former

Yugoslavia. This story deals with only one of the many types of torture and ethnic cleansing that occurred during the war. Other variations of this story dwell on forced sexual intercourse between parents and children, the witnessing of homosexual rape of males by their captors, and the rape of children by soldiers witnessed by parents (see chapter 1 vignette, "Rape Your Children or We Will Do It For You").

CASE EXAMPLE: "SERBIAN SPIT ROAST"

In telling her trauma story of abusive violence and war atrocities perpetrated against her family, a young Bosnian widow from Tuzla tearfully detailed an incident in which she was forced to watch her husband, bound and skewered on long metal rods, as he was burned alive on a "spit"—roasting apparatus while drunken Serbian soldiers laughed at his agonizing, tortured cries. During the frenzy of the Serbian massacre in 1995, the sadistic soldiers slowly turned the spit as his skin burned, and he lay "roasting" and dying at the hands of his captors. Held at gun point, the terrorized wife watched helplessly as her husband cried out in agony. Next, the intoxicated soldiers took turns raping the woman after her husband ceased his helpless pleas for mercy.

How can one hear such a story and not be psychically overwhelmed at the pure insanity of such a situation? How can the therapist not feel affect dysregulation and a loss of equilibrium? How does the therapist assist the bereaved woman in working through such traumatic memories?

This powerful trauma story makes salient the critical issue of empathic attunement versus empathic strains. How does one respond to the bereft, traumatized widow who was forced to watch her husband "spit-roasted" to death, and was then raped by her Serbian captors? How does one respond to her request to explain how God could allow such an atrocity? How does the therapist deal with his or her counteridentifications to this story? What is the critical role enactment sequence of the therapist at this point in TST? Is the role enactment that of the perpetrator? Of the protector? Of the helpless husband on the Serb's torture spit? Indeed, how does one maintain attunement and manifest empathic stretch?

Empathic stretch, a concept developed by Wilson and Lindy (1994), characterizes the internal working process of the therapist to keep the balance beam level between empathic strains and empathic attunement. Empathic stretch means that the therapists are forced, by the power of the trauma transference, to stretch and extend deeper into themselves, finding internal models, schemas, memories and emotional fortitude from their personal lives and professional experiences, to reach out as far as needed to create an *isochronous response*, one with *empathic congruence*, which resonates well enough to maintain a sensitively attuned therapeutic connection. In the strongest and most elemental sense, empathic stretch is the capacity to be fully present "in the moment" with the other person without fear, judgment or expectation. It is the relational process of knowledge of the therapist's state of being without uncentering, apprehension or anxiety and, by being able to communicate understanding of the journey of tribulation as guides, to assist in the process of gaining resolution. In essence, empathic stretch is a capacity to remain centered and grounded as therapists, accepting the reality and inherent humanness of patients' struggles to understand their immersion into the dark abyss of trauma.

REFERENCES

Campbell, J. (1949). *Hero with a thousand faces*. New York: Penguin Books.

Chu, J. A. (1999). *Rebuilding shattered lives: The responsible treatment of complex post-traumatic and dissociative disorders*. New York: Wiley.

Coen, S. (2002). *Affect intolerance in patient and analyst*. Northvale, NJ: Jason Aronson.

Courtois, C. (1999). *Recollections of sexual abuse: Treatment principles and guidelines*. New York: Norton.

Dalenberg, C. (2000). *Countertransference and PTSD*. Washington, DC: American Psychological Association Press.

Dalenberg, C. L. (2000). *Countertransference in the treatment of trauma*. Washington, DC: American Psychological Association Press.

Figley, C. R. (2002). *Treating compassion fatigue*. New York: Brunner-Routledge.

Foy, D. W., Schnurr, P. P., Weiss, D., Wattenberg, M. S., Glynn, S., Marmar, C. R. & Gusman, F. (2001). Group psychotherapy for PTSD. In J. P. Wilson, M. J. Friedman, & J. D. Lindy (Eds.), *Treating psychological trauma and PTSD* (pp. 183–205). New York: Guilford Publications.

Freud, S. (1917). *New introductory lectures on psychoanalysis*. New York: Norton.

Herman, J. (1992). *Trauma and recovery*. New York: Basic Books.

Horowitz, M. (1976). *Stress response syndromes*. Northvale, NJ: Jason Aronson.

Horowitz, M. (1986). *Stress response syndromes* (2nd ed.). Northvale, NJ: Jason Aronson.

Horowitz, M. (1993). Stress response syndromes: A review of posttraumatic and adjustment disorders. In J. P. Wilson & B. Raphael (Eds.), *International handbook of traumatic stress syndromes* (pp. 49–61). New York: Plenum Press.

LeDoux, J. E. (1996). *The emotional brain*. New York: Simon & Schuster.

Lindy, J. D. (1993). Focal psychoanalytic psychotherapy of PTSD. In J. P. Wilson & B. Raphael (Eds.), *International handbook of traumatic stress syndromes* (pp. 803–811). New York: Plenum Press.

McEwen, B. (1998). Protective and damaging effects of stress mediators. *Seminars of the Beth Israel Deaconess Medical Center, 338*(3), 171–179.

Parsons, E. (1988). Post-traumatic self-disorders. In J. P. Wilson, Z. Harel, & B. Kahana (Eds.), *Human adaptation to extreme stress: From the Holocaust to Vietnam* (pp. 245–279). New York: Plenum Press.

Parson, E. (1988). Theoretical and practical considerations in psychotherapy of Vietnam war veterans. In J. P. Wilson, Z. Harel, & B. Kahana (Eds.), *Human adaptation to extreme stress: From the Holocaust to Vietnam*. New York: Plenum Press.

Pearlman, L. & Saakvitne, K. (1995). *Trauma and the therapist*. New York: Norton.

Schore, A. N. (2003a). *Affect dysregulation and disorders of the self.* New York: Norton.

Schore, A. N. (2003b). *Affect regulation and the repair of the self.* New York: Norton.

Tansey, M. J. & Burke, W. F. (1989). *Understanding countertransference.* Hillsdale, NJ: Erlbaum.

Volkan, V. (2004). From hope to a better life to broken spirits. In J. P. Wilson & B. Drozdek (Eds.), *Broken spirits: The treatment of traumatized asylum seekers, refugees and war and torture victims.* New York: Brunner-Routledge.

Wilson, J. P. (2004). Broken spirits. In J. P. Wilson & B. Drozdek (Eds.), *Broken spirits: The treatment of traumatized asylum seekers, refugees and war and torture victims* (pp. 141–173). New York: Brunner-Routledge.

Wilson, J. P. & Drozdek, B. (2004). *Broken spirits: The treatment of traumatized asylum seekers, refugees and war and torture victims.* New York: Brunner-Routledge.

Wilson, J. P. Friedman, M. J., & Lindy, J. D. (2001). *Treating psychological trauma and PTSD.* New York: Guilford Publications.

Wilson, J. & Lindy, J. (1994). *Countertransference in the treatment of PTSD.* New York: Guilford Publications.

Zoellner, R., Fitzgibbons, L. A. & Foa, E. (2001). Cognitive behavioral approaches to PTSD. In J. P. Wilson, M. J. Friedman, & J. D. Lindy (Eds.), *Treating psychological trauma and PTSD* (pp. 159–183). New York: Guilford Publications.

4

A Model of Empathy in Trauma Work

Conceptualizing the intricate dynamics of empathy in trauma work requires a model that provides a "road map" to the component processes comprising the clinical nature of interactive phenomena between psychotherapists and their clients. A conceptual road map is a guide to the matrix of empathy, in the way an atlas marks a country's geographical regions. Figure 4.1 presents a model of the structure and dynamics of interpersonal processes in the treatment of PTSD. The model presents a magnified overview of the components of the empathic process and its "flow" of interactional sequences.

To begin, it is helpful to identify the key elements that constitute the model summarized in Figure 4.1. On the left-hand side of Figure 4.1 is a list of 10 categories of the structural dimensions of the model. For each of the 10 categories, corresponding categories which summarize the process variables are given on the right-hand side. To facilitate understanding of the overall structure of the model of empathic processes in trauma work, these 10 categories are studied in the discussion that follows. As the chapter develops, the role of empathy as presented in the model is analyzed, emphasizing how the processes of empathic strain and empathic attunement influence the therapist's capacity to manage trauma transference.

A MODEL OF EMPATHY IN TRAUMA WORK

The model of empathy in trauma work, given in Figure 4.1, is a schematic representation of a complex set of dynamic variables which influence the process of post-traumatic therapy. For example, the severity and nature of the client's traumatic state or PTSD is important to understand, as it influences the range of impacts it will have on the therapist. The therapist, in turn, needs to be able to decode trauma transference and the symbolic manifestations of traumatic experiences stored in implicit memory states. The nature of affective reactions experienced during the course of treatment has strong effects on empathic strains and empathic attunement, etc.

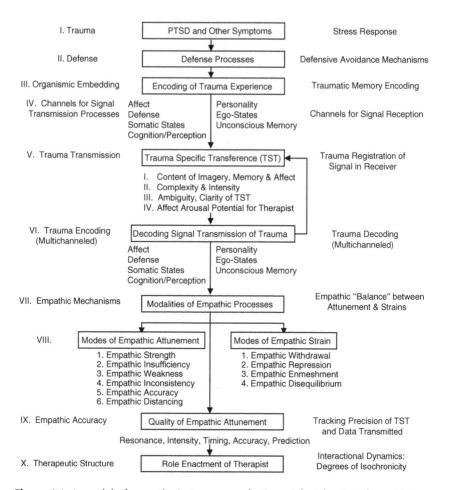

Figure 4.1 A model of empathy in trauma work. Copyright John P. Wilson, 2002.

For organizational purposes, each component of the model is discussed separately as foundational.

1. Trauma and Stress Response Patterns
2. Defense and Defensive Avoidance Mechanisms
3. Organismic Embedding and Traumatic Memory Encoding
4. Channels for Signal Transmission and Channels for Signal Reception
5. Trauma Transmission Processes and Trauma Registration of Signal in Receiver
6. Trauma Encoding (multichanneled) and Trauma Decoding (multi-channeled)

7. Empathic Mechanisms and Empathic Balance: Attunement Versus Strain
8. Modalities of Empathic Attunement and Modalities of Empathic Strain
9. Empathic Accuracy and Tracking Precision of TST and Data Transmission
10. Therapeutic Structure and Interactional Dynamics: Degrees of Isochronicity

TRAUMA, PTSD, CO-MORBIDITY AND PERSONALITY ALTERATIONS

A model of empathy in trauma work begins with an understanding of the complexities of post-traumatic states of traumatization. The patient with a history of trauma, especially early relational trauma (Schore, 2003a, 2003b), may manifest a wide range of psychological/psychiatric symptoms which include PTSD, other Axis I disorders, and significant alterations in personality processes that were not present prior to the trauma (Breslau, 1999; Kessler et al., 1995; Wilson, 2004; Wilson, Friedman, & Lindy, 2001). These post-traumatic changes in personality and behavioral dispositions reflect prolonged stress responses to trauma experiences. As discussed by McEwen (1998), Friedman (2001), and Wilson, Friedman, and Lindy (2001), prolonged stress responses are indicative of allostatic load wherein the organism creates a new "set point" of baseline functioning rather than returning to the homeostatic levels present before the trauma (see chapter 11 for a discussion).

By their nature, traumatic experiences cause injuries to physical and psychological integrity, wounding body, psyche and soul. When unresolved and persistent, the sequela of trauma alters organismic functioning at multiple system levels (e.g., memory, perceptual processes, attachment patterns, etc.) which get embedded in new psychological states created within the organism (Putnam, 1997). Since traumatic experiences are powerful and often overwhelming, they produce *affective dysregulations* in the brain and control systems that regulate emotions (LeDoux, 1996; Schore, 2003a, 2003b). Bruce McEwen (1998) has described these changes in the functioning of the sympathetic nervous system as allostasis, reflecting the dysregulation of cortical functions by extreme, repetitive or prolonged stress response tendencies.

At the psychological level, the sequela of prolonged stress response, especially in the form of PTSD, requires defensive attempts to protect the organism from the consequences produced by affective dysregulation, psychological disequilibrium and altered cognitive-behavioral states of adaptation (Putnam, 1997; Schore, 2003a, 2003b). The traumatized individual can only remain in an overdriven state of excessive arousal during the period before allostatic processes evoke significant psychological and health-related changes (Schnurr & Green, 2004). In this regard, empathy, as a process, includes the capacity to identify and understand disrupted psychological states produced by trauma.

DEFENSE AND ORGANISMIC MECHANISMS OF SECURITY AND PROTECTION

Trauma disrupts a person's sense of well-being, producing alterations at all levels of normal organismic functioning. These alterations take many forms which range from ego-defenses, such as dissociation, repression, denial, disavowal, suppression, projection, sublimation and altruism (Vaillant, 1999), to changes in worldview and systems of meaning and values. Ego-defenses attempt to bind anxiety, fears and states of psychological uncertainty which are typically associated with malaise, dysphoria, clinical symptoms of depression, and altered systems of meaning, values and beliefs about human nature. Ego-defenses and adaptive patterns of coping (Lazarus & Folkman, 1984) are among the cognitive processes associated with the initial (i.e., peri-traumatic) responses to trauma as well as prolonged attempts at processing the impact of trauma on organismic functioning.

The traumatic impact on organismic functioning involves powerful affective dysregulation, and results in relatively permanent changes in personality functioning which include the capacity to effectively regulate and monitor internal states. As Allan N. Schore (2003b) notes: "The fact that dissociation becomes a trait in post-traumatic stress disorders has devastating effects on the self, and therefore psychobiological functions" (p. 260). In this sense, the effects of trauma are embedded in the organism and represent the encoding of the trauma experience. A model of empathy needs to promote an understanding of the function of ego- and organismic mechanisms of defensive security and protection which are set in motion by the traumatic injury. These processes constitute the second element in the model. Trauma mars the whole person; its effects are not restricted to the site of injury—be it a broken leg or a combat scarred psyche.

ORGANISMIC EMBEDDING OF TRAUMA

In terms of holistic functioning, it is important to understand that traumatic experiences are embedded organismically in subsystems with their own command and control functions (Friedman, 2000; Wilson, 2004). Part III of the model indicates that, as part of an integrated psychobiological system, traumatic experiences have cascade effects across various brain and neurohormonal mechanisms which comprise the infrastructure of prolonged stress responses (Friedman, 2000). As Figure 4.1 illustrates, the encoding of the trauma experience occurs at multiple levels which have different pathways of expression in behavior. These different pathways are channels for *signal transmissions* by the patient of the status of organismic functioning at any given point in time.

As noted in chapter 1, there are seven primary channels by which the state of organismic disequilibrium caused by trauma gets expressed, including as a function of PTSD: (1) affect; (2) defenses; (3) somatic states; (4) cognitive and perceptual processes; (5) personality; (6) ego-states; and (7) unconscious processes, including unconscious memory. The encoding of the trauma experience within the organism means that expressions of altered psychobiological states are transmitted in various ways, in terms of perception, memory, defense, adaptation and coping. Parts IV, V and VI of the model represent the encoding, storage and transmission of information about traumatized psychic and organismic states.

In post-traumatic therapy, the organismically embedded information associated with the trauma experience will most likely be evident in TST reactions throughout the course of treatment (Wilson & Lindy, 1994). TST reactions are those behaviors manifested by a patient that are associated with unmetabolized elements of the traumatic event, and involve symbolic and other forms of reenactment with the therapist. TST reactions are projections of ego- and organismic states of adjustment which may also be encoded in any of the seven channels for transmission. As indicated in chapter 1, TST projections emanating from the patient can be considered in different ways which include such descriptions as *flow, waves, signals, energy, information, transmissions, postural freezing, archetypal configurations,* and *masks of trauma* in the persona of personality (Wilson, 2004).

By its very nature, TST is a complex phenomenon, one in which the patient's unconscious sends encoded messages to the therapist. It is the process of empathic attunement which enables precise and accurate decoding of the information being transmitted in multichanneled ways by the patient to the therapist. As noted by Wilson and Lindy (1994), TST reactions have four primary dimensions: (1) the content of images, traumatic memory and affects; (2) the complexity and intensity of the information being transmitted; (3) the clarity or ambiguity of the signal transmission of trauma-related material; and (4) the affect arousal potential (AAP) of the traumatic narrative for the therapist. The impact of TST on the therapist may be subtle or overwhelmingly forceful, generating powerful visceral effects within the therapist while listening to the accounts of individual trauma experiences. Illustrative of this point is the strong emotions evoked by a perusal of the case vignettes presented at the beginning of chapter 1, leading some readers to skip head to other chapters in this book or simply put it down and stop reading it altogether.

TRAUMA TRANSMISSION AND TRAUMA SPECIFIC TRANSFERENCE REACTIONS

The organismic encoding of psychological trauma is registered in implicit memory. As Jean Knox (2003) notes,

> In essence, it is the concepts of implicit memory and the internal working model which provide the basis for a paradigm shift in relation to our understanding of the human psyche; if information is inaccessible to the consciousness, not because it is actively repressed but simply because it is encoded and stored in a format that is unavailable to consciousness, then the idea that such material can be made conscious by the analyst's interpretation which overcomes repression, is doomed to failure. (p. 181)

This insight is especially useful in understanding TST as a manifestation of altered organismic and ego-states of being. Knox (2003) suggests that powerful emotional experiences, especially those with attachment figures, can be

> actively resolved in the present relationship with the analyst, usually without awareness that the present experience is being distorted by powerful patterns of expectations and emotions which form a key part of the activated implicit memories. (p. 181)

In TST reactions, the patient tends to focus on the specific elements (e.g., images, thoughts, fragmented memories, dreams, etc.) concerned with the dynamics that occurred during the traumatic event. These experiences are stored in both the explicit and the implicit memory, the latter being more state-dependent and less accessible to complete conscious recall (Putnam, 1997). Nevertheless, in TST, the patient transmits, in multichanneled ways, cues to the contents of the trauma experience, partly by the trauma narrative and partly through allusion to implicit memories which encapsulate painful aspects of the traumatic episode. Through the process of TST projections (i.e., transmissions of data about how the experience is encoded in memory), the patient necessarily places the therapist in *trauma specific roles* which have important meaning and significance due to the nature of the transference. For example, depending on the type of trauma experienced, a therapist could be cast into the role enactment of a seductive perpetrator (sexual abuse), demonic torturer (political oppression), fellow combatant (military stressors), indifferent parental figures (familial neglect), or fellow survivor (political internment). In this manner, then, there is an *isomorphism* in TST; over time, the patient reenacts, in the therapeutic setting, specific aspects of the trauma experience(s).

Moreover, with the establishment of a safe therapeutic sanctuary and a good working alliance, the contents of trauma-related imagery, memories and affects will unfold of their own accord, with varying levels of affective intensity and capacity to impact the therapist's sense of stability, control, and clarity in understanding the process itself. It is precisely at this point that the capacity to sustain empathic attunement is critical, since the task of decoding TST and other forms of transference is contingent upon the precision of attunement in the process of understanding, decoding transmissions, and interpretation. As discussed later, isochronous, concordant and synchronized empathic interchange permits a healthy resonance between patient and therapist. Empathic congruence by the therapist to the client's TST presentations promotes "organismic tuning," the reduction of negative allostatic stress load and the facilitation of positive allostatic changes towards restabilization and optimal levels of adaptive functioning (see chapter 11). To sustain empathic attunement requires the capacity to decode signal transmissions associated with implicit memory, state-dependent information and the ability to develop a holistic gestalt of the patient's trauma experience.

DECODING SIGNAL TRANSMISSIONS OF TRAUMA

The art of interpreting the dynamics of a traumatized client is challenging, difficult and frequently fraught with impasses during the course of treatment. In its simplest and perhaps purest form, the task of interpretation involves assisting clients in understanding their own internalized working models of the trauma experience, and the formation of new perspectives and ways of understanding how the trauma impacted their personality and adaptive coping efforts (Everly & Lating, 2003).

Empathic attunement is a primary vehicle in this effort, enabling the therapist to decode the patient's "signal transmissions" in any of the seven primary channels. Traumatic memory reflects how the trauma experience was encoded in explicit and implicit forms of memory (Putnam, 1997; van der Kolk, 1999). The patient's capacity to report these internal states is governed, to a large extent, by control processes (e.g., defenses) which regulate the manner in which trauma is processed at conscious and unconscious levels by the patient. Thus, decoding and interpretation are interrelated dynamically during the course of post-traumatic treatment. However, decoding is the therapist's task to understand, as precisely as possible, how the internal working model reflects the patient's cognitive schema. It is for this reason, then, that the process of decoding underlies the modalities of empathic attunement and empathic strain.

MODALITIES OF EMPATHIC FUNCTIONING

The quality of empathic functioning in the course of post-traumatic treatment is a dynamic, fluctuating and variable effective process. Parts VII through IX in the model identify the key processes concerned with the matrix of empathy and the quality of empathic functioning. During treatment sessions the degrees of empathic attunement range from minimal to optimal. Empathic attunement can be conceptualized as a process, an ability or the capacity of the analyst. Empathic attunement also exists on a scalable continuum, ranging from detachment and disengagement to optimal states of accurate empathic resonance. In this sense, the empathic continuum and modes of empathic attunement can be thought of as ranging from optimal states of effective, functional connections with clients' transmissions of their concerns and current life issues, to states of separation, withdrawal, distance, dissociation, detachment and minimal or nonfunctional connectedness to the internal working model of the patient's trauma experience.

As a third level of analysis, the continuum of empathic functioning also underlies the continuum of CTRs described by Wilson and Lindy (1994). Minimal empathic attunement, characterized by detachment, disengagement, withdrawal, avoidance and inadequate decoding of TST comprises a part of Type I countertransference modality: *avoidance reactions*. In contrast, optimal empathic attunement is characterized by decoding accuracy, effective and functional styles of patient engagement which, in some cases, leads to overidentification and idealization of the patient with Type II CTRs: *overidentification*.

MODES OF EMPATHIC ATTUNEMENT AND EMPATHIC STRAIN

Empathic attunement and empathic strain are interrelated dimensions of empathic responding. (Chapter 5 discusses the problem of maintaining balance between the two modalities as the problem of the "balance beam" in sustaining empathic attunement.) Empathic attunement defines individual ability to effectively use empathy during the course of treatment. As described by Kohut (1977), empathy is a means of understanding and knowing about a patient's individual experiences. In this respect, empathy, as a process, is a vehicle to obtaining useful information about the data provided by the patient. Empathic attunement is accurate resonance; it is a good interconnection between therapist and patient which is isochronous in nature, manifesting states of coevality, synchronization, coetaneous matching responses and response concordance. The opposite of empathic attunement is empathic separation and detachment, usually caused by factors that strain the therapist's capacity for sustaining empathic attunement.

Empathic strains are disruptive processes which interfere with the therapist's ability to sustain empathic inquiry; to maintain empathic accuracy in decoding signal transmissions from the patient, including TST;

and to form the basis of CTRs. Wilson and Lindy (1994) define empathic strain as "interpersonal [or intrapersonal] events in psychotherapy that weaken, injure, or force beyond due limits a salutary response to a client" (p. 27).

The many potential sources of empathic strain in work with PTSD clients include: (1) affective dysregulation in the therapist while listening to powerful and emotionally intense trauma histories; (2) cognitive disillusionment induced in the therapist by confronting the realities of human cruelty, malevolence, capacity for aggression, willful infliction of pain and suffering as well as neglect, emotional indifference and unbridled and ruthless egoism; (3) the subtleties and intricate nuances of TST, in which the therapist is cast into various roles (e.g., judge, lover, perpetrator) which may be uncomfortable to realize and manage therapeutically; (4) the constancy of omnipresent, affectively dysregulated states in the trauma patient which tax the therapist's coping strength and lead to fatigue; (5) the power of trauma stories to reactivate areas of personal vulnerability in the therapist, including unresolved issues of childhood development; (6) the lack of education and training in traumatic stress, PTSD, stress disorders and inadequate knowledge of the syndrome dynamics of PTSD (Wilson, 2004); (7) rigid, ideological adherence to a specific school of psychotherapy and intellectual dogmatism in respect of PTSD as a fixed entity, as an anxiety disorder rather than a dynamic, fluctuating state of prolonged stress with many allostatic variations which influence symptom production, self-presentations and somatic processes at any given time (McEwen, 1998; Wilson, 2004; Wilson, Friedman, & Lindy, 2001).

Figure 4.1 indicates six modes of empathic attunement and four modes of empathic strain. These processes are two sides of a coin: they coexist, affecting the quality of empathic accuracy, proper attunement and connection to the patient's signal transmissions. The maintenance of good empathic resonance results in empathic congruence, isochronicity and "response matching" between therapist and patient. Empathic strain can result in ineffective therapist responsiveness, inadequate signal decoding, and states of tense separation between patient and therapist which could result in either a Type I or Type II CTR. The twin modes of empathic attunement and empathic strain directly affect the qualities of empathic attunement which contain six dimensions: (i) resonance; (ii) intensity; (iii) timing; (iv) accuracy; (v) prediction; and (vi) isochronicity.

QUALITIES OF EMPATHIC ATTUNEMENT IN TRAUMA WORK

Empathic attunement is the ability to respond optimally with accuracy in understanding the internal working model of the client's trauma

I.	**Resonance:** resonance, synchrony and being "in phase" with the patient's internal state, specifically as it pertains to the trauma experience and trauma story
II.	**Intensity:** affect modulation in which the level of intensity is understood, received and processed without distortion
III.	**Timing:** responsiveness (i.e., communicative cadence) which demonstrates phasic synchrony with the patient's ego-state and internal level of affect arousal
IV.	**Accuracy:** the precision of decoding, knowing or inferring the patient's internal psychological state
V.	**Prediction:** the ability to extrapolate and accurately predict future behavioral patterns and dynamics of the patients
VI.	**Isochronicity:** the overall synchronicity, flow, "in-beat" capacity to respond relatively consistently with the patient's internal model encoded, pathogenic and non-pathogenic schema

Note: All six qualities are operational and capable of empirical quantification (see Stern, 1985).

Figure 4.2 Qualities* of empathic attunement in trauma work. Copyright John P. Wilson, 2002.

experience. Optimal empathic attunement is characterized by proper timing, good affect modulation in the therapist, accuracy in decoding signals and TST, and the maintenance of isochronous functioning. It is resonant, "in-the-beat," and has phasic synchronicity with the patient. The qualities of empathic attunement (see Figure 4.2) include (i) *resonance,* or being in phase with the patient's internal state; (ii) *intensity,* that is, the capacity for affect modulation by the therapist which does not lead to empathic strains; (iii) *timing,* that is, appropriate timing of responsiveness which demonstrates phasic synchrony with the client's ego-states and levels of affect arousal; (iv) *accuracy,* or the degree of precision in decoding and knowing the patient's internal psychological state; (v) *prediction,* or the ability to accurately predict the client's future behavioral patterns; and (vi) *isochronicity,* that is, the overall empathic congruence and phasic synchronicity, over time, with the internal state of the working model of the trauma experience.

EVOLVING THERAPEUTIC STRUCTURE AND INTERACTIONAL DYNAMICS

The model of empathy in trauma work is a schema of the structure and dynamics of interpersonal processes in the treatment of PTSD. It describes a flow of psychological interactions between patient and therapist. Figure 4.1 indicates that the outcome of the operation of empathy is the evolution, over time, of a therapeutic structure that emerges from the interactional dynamics of the treatment process (see part X of the model). As a structural variable, empathy has unique dimensions, including the emergent nature of role differentiation in a dyadic relationship (Aronoff & Wilson, 1985). More specifically, this evolved role of differentiation includes the various role enactments into which the therapist is placed by transference dynamics.

Carl G. Jung (1963) was among the first analysts to recognize empathic mutuality as indigenous to analytic work. He observed that the therapist, by willingly receiving the patient's anxiety, pain, conflicts, traumas and human struggles, could also be wounded in the process:

> For since the analytical work must inevitably lead sooner or later to a fundamental discussion between "I" and "you" and "you" and "I" on a plane stripped of all human pretenses, it is very likely, indeed almost certain, that not only the patient but the doctor as well will find the situation *"getting under his skin."* Nobody can *meddle with fire or poison* without being affected in some vulnerable spot; for the true physician does not stand outside his work but always is in the thick of it. (p. 131)

This quote from Jung is instructive because it highlights the mutuality of the therapeutic process; both patient and analyst are affected in different and, sometimes, similar ways. Further, since the "advent" of PTSD as a focus of scientific study and clinical inquiry, researchers have developed terms to characterize both sides of the analytic situation. For example, the impact of the PTSD patient on the therapist has been referred to as vicarious traumatization (Pearlman & Saakvitne, 1995), compassion fatigue (Figley, 1995), empathic distress (Wilson & Lindy, 1994), secondary traumatic stress reaction, helper stress, burnout, emotional contagion and borrowed stress (Figley, 2002). These terms reflect efforts to understand the processes we have identified in the model, and underscore the fact that dealing with traumatized persons is hard work, requiring perseverance, stamina, emotional balance, knowledge of prolonged traumatic stress responses, clinical insight and experience. These same terms describe the therapist's reactions to work with traumatized persons—all reactions share the core component of identifying stressful impacts on the mental health professional.

The larger issue, however, is not whether post-traumatic therapy is inherently difficult and replete with risk factors, but how these factors exert a reciprocal influence on the success of therapists' efforts to help those afflicted by traumatic life experiences. As Jung (1944, 1951) observed, an empathic mutuality exists in which there is an array of dynamics at work in the treatment process. For this reason, understanding of traumatized states, including PTSD, is paramount. The moot question is: what are the core factors that influence empathic orientation and the capacity for empathic attunement?

FACTORS INFLUENCING EMPATHIC ORIENTATION

Figure 4.3 presents a summary of the core variables that influence empathic orientation during post-traumatic therapy. These five factors have been reviewed by Ervin Staub (1979) in his classic two-volume work, *Positive Social Behavior and Morality*. As Figure 4.3 illustrates, a person with good social skills, advanced moral development, strong ego-strength, and genetic/temperamental disposition for empathic ability may be expected to have a natural propensity for empathic attunement with others. Similarly, we may presume that persons with a history of psychological trauma would be sensitive to cues of affective distress, anxiety, dissociative states and symptoms of PTSD. We may likewise expect a person with a broad range of life experiences to have more empathic strength, given the exposure to diversity of culture, and the awareness of universal human struggles in life. As conceived more inclusively, these five factors (developmental level, ego-strength, trauma history, life experience and psychobiological attunement capacity) can be considered as dispositional

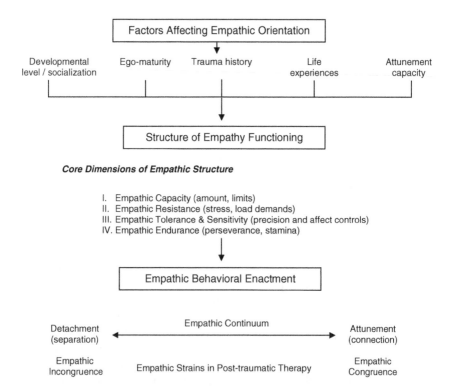

Figure 4.3 Factors influencing empathic orientation. Copyright John P. Wilson, 2002.

variables which underpin the structure of empathic functioning (see chapter 9 for empirical data on these issues).

CORE DIMENSIONS OF EMPATHIC STRUCTURE: CAPACITY, RESISTANCE, TOLERANCE AND ENDURANCE

As Figure 4.3 and 4.4 illustrate, it is possible to define a clinically meaningful continuum of empathic functioning. This continuum ranges from a minimal level (detachment, disengagement) to optimal levels (attunement, engagement). It is also possible to conceptualize this continuum as ranging from degrees of empathic separation to empathic connection. *Empathic separation* is characterized as minimally effective functioning, with insufficiencies in decoding signal transmissions from the patient in

Basic Dispositions: Empathic Attunement vs. Empathic Separation and Detachment
A. Attunement: receptive, good matching, accurate resonance, minimal distortion/interference
B. Separation: receptive blocks, interference, inadequate matching, inaccurate resonance, distortion, "noise," interference

EMPATHIC DIMENSIONS

I. **Empathic Capacity**

A.   Amount and limits of system capacity to maintain fundamental attunement

B.   Capacity is determined by genetics, personality and experience in trauma work

II. **Empathic Resistance**

A.   Amount of capacity of system to resist being overloaded by stress demands

B.   Resistance associated with four factors: (1) trauma story; (2) personal factors in therapist; (3) institutional constraints on resources; and (4) personal factors in patient (gender, age, race, type of trauma)

III. **Empathic Tolerance & Sensitivity**

A.   Amount of system tolerance capacity in response to demands that challenge accuracy of empathic attunement capacity (i.e., allostatic load capacity)

B.   Sensitivity to precision of empathic congruency and tolerance in capacity to control personal tensions while maintaining sensitivity and attunement to patient

IV. **Empathic Endurance**

A.   Degree of perseverance and sustainability (stamina) in the process of maintaining empathic attunement

B.   Endurance capacity directly correlated with psychological wellbeing of the therapist

Figure 4.4 Dimensions of empathic functioning: A continuum of attunement to separation and detachment. Copyright John P. Wilson, 2002.

the form of verbal, nonverbal and transference projections, including TST (Wilson & Lindy, 1994). *Empathic attunement*, in contrast, is maximally effective in decoding signal (informational) transmission from the patient to the therapist.

The four core dimensions of the structure of empathy need to be defined in terms of their relationship to the outcome of psychotherapy. These four dimensions are interrelated but independent factors, exerting a powerful influence on the operation of empathy in the interpersonal dynamics of clinical treatment, which includes medical settings, crisis debriefings, psychotherapy and research studies involving face-to-face protocol administration and/or psychological assessments (Wilson & Keane, 2004).

Empathic capacity specifically refers to the proficiency and limits of the therapist in maintaining an attitude of empathic attunement. Empathic capacity can be conceptualized as the ability of the "system" to respond efficaciously across different clinical settings, social interactions and diverse situations in which empathic capacity could serve as a tool for information retrieval, processing and understanding. *Empathic endurance* is associated with empathic capacity but indicates the degree of perseverance and sustainability of empathic attunement. We assume that empathic endurance is correlated with the psychological well-being of the psychotherapist. *Empathic sensitivity and empathic tolerance* are interrelated aspects of the core dimensions of empathy. *Empathic sensitivity* connotes the precision of empathic attunement. How well "tuned-in" is the therapist to the patient? Sensitivity also signifies the capacity to identify different frequencies and strengths of signal transmissions from the patient. A highly sensitive "receiver" can detect many signal frequencies with precision, even if the strength of the signal is weak. This can be construed as a *multichanneled sensitivity* which, in terms of post-traumatic therapies, means that the clinicians can "read," "understand," "register," "decide on" or "receive" a wide spectrum of trauma specific cues (TSC) emanating from the patient. These cues, especially TSCs, may be verbal, nonverbal, nested in fantasy, dreams or free associations (Kalsched, 2003; Knox, 2003).

However, irrespective of the source, a set of informational transmissions from the patient (e.g., the trauma narrative; childhood developmental history; etc.) is assumed to contain relevant material that can be empathically understood through attunement, leading to useful and interpretable material (i.e., decoded data from the transference projection). Therefore, *empathic tolerance* refers to the capacity of the system to tolerate demands for accurate "signal detection" in information transmissions from the patient. In extreme situations, the patient's affective intensity (e.g., anger, rage, suicidal tendency, traumatic bereavement) may be multichanneled and acute at the same time, presenting the clinician with a complexity of dense data in the form of feelings, narratives, moral dilemmas, and impossible choices in the midst of the client's traumatic experience. In such situations, patients exude affective intensity (e.g., rage, profound sorrow), and pour out condensed or splintered accounts of their overwhelming experiences which may be difficult to track, decode, tune in on the proper frequency, or monitor multichanneled messages and units of personal data encoded in their memory. These encoded memories are part of the internal working model of the patient's experiences and may not be adequately processed into existing cognitive schema (Knox, 2003). The transmission of this information may appear garbled, unclear, fragmented, incoherent or confusing. This multi-channeled set of data is important as a structural form with meaning, and in terms of its discernible affective intensity. As an overall structural form or configuration of an informational signal process, it is akin to the patient saying: "Look, there is so much I want to tell you, but it's so overwhelming that I cannot express all of it at once very well." This ambiguity and *informational density* may tax the therapist's capacity for empathic tolerance.

Empathic tolerance is the capacity to contain such multichanneled TST projections from patients with PTSD, and to sustain empathic attunement in the face of high demands (i.e., allostatic stress loads). In this sense, *empathic tolerance* is a variant on the therapist's capacity to adequately modulate allostatic stress loads to challenged levels of optimal functioning. The moderating factor of empathic tolerance is the feature of *empathic resistance*, which is defined as the capacity of the system to resist being overloaded, and losing signal detection ability imposed by load

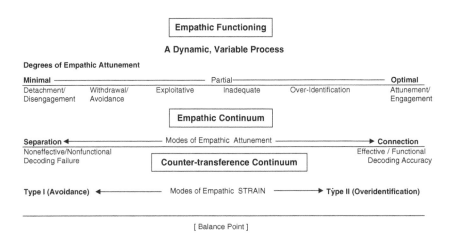

Figure 4.5 Continuum of empathic functioning: Detachment versus attunement. Copyright John P. Wilson, 2002.

demands. As noted by Wilson and Lindy (1994), empathic resistance (i.e., the capacity to weather attacks on empathic attunement) is associated with four factors which can lead to empathic strains on optimal effectiveness: (i) trauma story; (ii) personal factors; (iii) client factors; and (iv) organizational constraints. *Empathic resistance* is the system's capacity, akin to that of a resistor in electronics, to modulate the "flow" of energy within the system to ensure optimal functioning. However, with excessive demand and overload, empathic resistance may fail, resulting in a rupture of empathy and one of the many forms of countertransference possible in post-traumatic psychotherapy. Figure 4.5 illustrates the continuum of countertransference modalities which is discussed more fully in chapter 5.

REFERENCES

Aronoff, J. & Wilson, J. P. (1985). *Personality in the social process.* Livingston, NJ: Erlbaum.

Breslau, N. (1999). Psychological trauma, epidemiology of trauma and PTSD. In R. Yehuda (Ed.), *Psychological trauma, epidemiology of trauma and posttraumatic stress disorder* (pp. 1–27). Washington, DC: American Psychiatric Press.

Everly, G. & Lating, J. (2003). *Personality guided therapy for posttraumatic stress disorders.* Washington, DC: American Psychological Association.

Figley, C. R. (1995). *Compassion fatigue.* New York: Brunner/Mazel.

Figley, C. R. (2002). *Treating compassion fatigue.* New York: Brunner-Routledge.

Friedman, M. J. (2000). *Posttraumatic and acute stress disorders.* Kansas City, MO: Compact Clinicals.

Friedman, M. J. (2000). *Post-traumatic stress disorder: The latest assessment and treatment strategies.* Kansas City, MO: Compact Clinicals.

Friedman, M. J. (2001). Allostatic versus empirical perspectives on pharmacotherapy. In J. P. Wilson, M. J. Friedman, & J. D. Lindy (Eds.), *Treating psychological trauma and PTSD* (pp. 94–125). New York: Guilford Publications.

Jung, C. G. (1929). The therapeutic value of abreaction (H. Read, M. Fordham, & G. Adler, Eds., Vol. 16). In *Collected works of C. J. Jung* (Vols. 1–20, R. F. C. Hull, Trans.). Princeton, NJ: Princeton University Press.

Jung, C. G. (1953–1979). *Collected works of C. J. Jung* (Vols. 1–20, R. F. C. Hull, Trans.). Princeton, NJ: Princeton University Press.

Jung, C. G. (1963). *Memories, dreams and reflections.* New York: Vintage Books.

Kalsched, D. (2003). Daimonic elements in early trauma. *Journal of Analytical Psychology, 48*(2), 145–176.

Kessler, R. C., Sonnega, A., Bromet, E., Hughes, M. H. & Nelson, C. B. (1995). Posttraumatic stress disorder in the national comorbidity survey. *Archives of General Psychiatry, 52,* 1048–1060.

Knox, J. (2003). *Archetype, attachment, analysis.* London: Brunner-Routledge.

Kohut, H. (1977). *The restoration of the self.* New York: International Universities Press.

Lazarus, R. & Folkman, S. (1984). *Stress, appraisal and coping.* New York: Springer.

LeDoux, J. E. (1996). *The emotional brain.* New York: Simon & Schuster.

McEwen, B. (1998). Protective and damaging effects of stress mediators. *Seminars of the Beth Israel Deaconess Medical Center, 338*(3), 171–179.

Pearlman, L. & Saakvitne, K. (1995). *Trauma and the therapist.* New York: Norton.

Putnam, F. (1997). *Dissociation in children and adolescents.* New York: Guilford Publications.

Schnurr, P. P. & Green, B. L. (2004). *Trauma and health: Physical consequences of exposure to extreme stress*. Washington, DC: American Psychological Association.

Schore, A. N. (2003a). *Affect dysregulation and disorders of the self*. New York: Norton.

Schore, A. N. (2003b). *Affect regulation and the repair of the self*. New York: Norton.

Staub, E. (1979). *Positive social behavior and morality*. New York: Academic Press.

Vaillant, G. (1999). *The wisdom of the ego*. New York: Norton.

Van der Kolk, B. (1999). The body keeps score: Memory and the evolving psychobiology of posttraumatic stress. In M. Horowitz (Ed.), *Essential papers on posttraumatic stress disorder* (pp. 301–327). New York: New York University Press.

Wilson, J. P. (2004). The broken spirit: Posttraumatic damage to the self. In J. P. Wilson & B. Drozdek (Eds.), *Broken spirits: The treatment of traumatized asylum seekers, refugees and war and torture victims* (pp. 107–155). New York: Brunner-Routledge.

Wilson, J. P. (2004). Broken spirits. In J. P. Wilson & B. Drozdek (Eds.), *Broken spirits: The treatment of traumatized asylum seekers, refugees and war and torture victims*. New York: Brunner-Routledge.

Wilson, J. P. & Drozdek, B. (2004). *Broken spirits: The treatment of traumatized asylum seekers, refugees and war and torture victims*. New York: Brumer-Routledge.

Wilson, J. P., Friedman, M. J. & Lindy, J. D. (2001). *Treating psychological trauma and PTSD*. New York: Guilford Publications.

Wilson, J. P. & Keane, T. M. (2004). *Assessing psychological trauma and PTSD* (2nd ed.). New York: Guilford Publications.

Wilson, J. & Lindy, J. (1994). *Countertransference in the treatment of PTSD*. New York: Guilford Publications.

5

The Balance Beam: Modes of Empathic Attunement and Empathic Strain in Post-Traumatic Therapy

> Therapeutic empathy requires a careful and attentive listener…it is not only the patient who must be perceived, but voices that emanate from within the therapist as well.
>
> *The Empathic Healer: An Endangered Species* (Bennett, 2001, p. 16)

Empathy is a tool for understanding the inner world of the psyche and soul of traumatized individuals. Empathy is a means of entry into injured spaces in the ego and spirit of persons suffering from PTSD, as well as into the abyss of the unconscious which is overwrought by trauma experiences. Empathic resonance of the highest caliber has the potential to unlock closed chambers in which the ego has sealed away overwhelmingly frightening experiences. Heinz Kohut (1982) believes that good psychotherapeutic interpretation goes "from a lower form to a higher form of empathy" (p. 395). Implicit in this appraisal of clinical activity is the idea that "higher forms" of empathy are more effective in treatment in terms of understanding and interpreting of material from the client.

The foregoing assessment raises important questions. What defines higher empathy? What is it about higher forms of empathy that makes therapeutic interpretations more useful, "on target" and facilitative of the patient's acceptance and use in integrating emotionally troublesome experiences? How does the therapist achieve higher empathic skills? How does the therapist, treating traumatized persons suffering from PTSD, depression, anxiety states and injuries to the self, maintain balance in the face of emotionally laden trauma stories? How does the therapist walk the balance beam between empathic attunement and empathic strain?

BRIEF HISTORICAL PERSPECTIVE OF EMPATHY AND PSYCHODYNAMIC THERAPY

The relationship between empathy, countertransference processes and mechanisms of identification by the patient or the therapist (counteridentification) has emerged in thoughtful and critical reviews in psychoanalytic literature. We will discuss some of the major literature reviews to illustrate the pattern of reemergence of the significance of empathy to countertransference, analytical interpretations, and intrapsychic thoughts and affects in the therapist.

In his comprehensive treatise, *Countertransference*, Edmond Slakter (1987) reviewed the psychoanalytic views on countertransference "from Freud's original remarks in 1910 to current views" (p. 3). This interesting and informative critique includes a chapter entitled "Countertransference and Empathy," in which the author expresses his own views on countertransference after concluding his review of psychoanalytic literature.

> In almost every analysis, empathy and countertransference seem so entwined that it is difficult to separate them. Are they in fact *separate phenomena*? *It is my belief that they are and that part of the analyst's task in treatment is to untangle them and clarify their relationship to each other.* (p. 201, italics ours)

This statement reflects Slakter's belief that empathy and countertransference are distinct processes and must be "untangled" in the course of treatment. He continues by defining empathy:

> Empathy is one person's partial identification with another person. In the therapeutic situation, the analyst's empathy consists of his ability to project his own personality onto that of the patient in order to understand him better. As is implied in this definition, empathy is partly a counter-transferential reaction. (p. 201)

This passage hints at the fact that Slakter sees empathy as a vehicle of understanding through "identification" with the patient, and therefore empathy is "partly" a process of countertransference. However, what does identification as a process mean? What, precisely, is the nature of such a process of identification? If empathy is only partly a "countertransference reaction," what else is it? What constitutes other empathic processes? Slakter provides a partial answer to these questions:

> An important link between empathy and countertransference is counteridentification, whereby the analyst both identifies with the patient and at the same time pulls back from that identification so as to view the patient with objectivity. Empathy is based on counter-identification; indeed, it is counter-identification that permits our empathy to be therapeutically useful. But,

counter-identification is also a component of countertransference, and if *it operates imperfectly, whereby objectivity is not achieved, then the analyst's negative countertransference reactions can cause his empathy to diminish or even vanish altogether.* When this happens, he may become *vulnerable* to additional negative *countertransference reactions.* And if then, in turn, he fails to analyze them, may lead to countertransference *acting out.* (p. 203, italics ours)

This statement by Slakter is quite similar to the analyses of others (e.g., Hedges, 1992) who have explored the dynamics of the interrelationships between empathy, identification processes and countertransference. As we have highlighted, Slakter hints at the problem of the balance beam: how to maintain empathic attunement when challenged by the stresses and strains indigenous to analytic treatment approaches. He correctly notes that "imperfect" empathy or counteridentification based on empathy, may lead "empathy to diminish ... or vanish," or may result in "acting out" of unmetabolized countertransference issues. Insufficient empathy, empathic failure or the total loss of empathic attunement has a range of potentially adverse, counterproductive, disruptive and potentially pathogenic consequences for treatment. This being the case, we can ask: How is it that empathic attunement is sustained? What set of criteria define empathic attunement, resonance and what Kohut referred to as "higher empathy"? What are the dimensions and characteristics of "higher empathy"?

The issue of the dimensions of empathy and their relationship has been explored in psychoanalytic writings. In a thoughtful critique which attempts to develop a model synthesizing disparate positions on the issue, Tansey and Burke (1989) in their book, *Understanding Countertransference,* state that

the operations of empathy and projective identification have traditionally been differentiated with respect to four characteristics: the *intense versus mild impact* on the therapist, the *intrapsychic versus interpersonal* nature of the process, *pathology versus normality,* and therapist's degree of conscious *control versus unconscious reactiveness* to experience. (p. 60, italics ours)

Tansey and Burke identify four distinguishing categories involving empathy and projective identification: (1) *relational,* that is, interpersonal versus intrapsychic; (2) *affect level,* that is, intense versus mild; (3) *awareness,* that is, conscious versus unconscious; and (4) *quality,* that is, normal versus pathological. The authors suggest that these four factors are at work during the therapeutic process and exert dynamic influences on the levels of empathic attunement that make this possible. For example, if a therapist were to experience intense affect caused by a difficult patient's behavior which rekindled unresolved character pathology in the analyst, we would assume that empathy and the quality of the identification process would be less than under optimal conditions. Tansey and Burke seem to be in agreement with this conclusion and state,

> Under optimal conditions in the empathic sequence, the therapist, having allowed the *interactional pressure to unfold within workable limits,* has interactional experience characterized by particular self-experiences and their associated *affective states.* The therapist can be thought of as having introjected a communication that exerts a modifying influence on his experiences of self in interaction. His *affective reaction* to the particular self-experience elicited by the immediate interaction optimally is signal affect... (p. 81, italics ours)

We can see that Tansey and Burke are proposing that affective states and their "signal" messages provide clues as to whether or not good identification with the patient has been made. They further assume that clarity and usefulness of *"signal affect"* occur when the therapist's capacity to receive the information is "within tolerable and reasonable limits" (p. 82) and that, when such optimal conditions exist, there is enhanced awareness in the therapist.

What if the therapist's capacity, due to the sheer intensity of TST, for example, is not within tolerable limits? What if sub-optimal conditions exist, in which there is such *low* intensity (e.g., therapist boredom, preoccupation, drowsiness, sleepiness) or *extreme* intensity (e.g., fear, overwhelmed states, profound sadness) that the "signal affects" overwhelm conscious awareness and the capacity to process the information being generated. Stated metaphorically, what if the "signal affects" blow out the "central processing unit" of the therapist? How then does empathic attunement get restored when empathic strains have caused the therapist to "fall off" the balance beam?

In their summary analysis, Tansey and Burke (1989) state,

> all successful processing of projective identifications will ultimately result in concordant empathic knowledge [cf. attunement] of the patient...Our knowledge of projective identification and empathy contradicts the notion that they are congruent and individually based operations, with the therapist engaging in empathy and the patient engaging in projective identification. *We understand both patient and therapist to be mutually involved in the operation of projective identification....* . Finally, the patient interaction working model implies that the therapist listens to the patient's material as if the therapist were the patient. (pp. 196–197, 203, italics ours)

Tansey and Burke have emphasized the relational dynamics concerning empathy, projective identification and its relation to "affect signals" in the communication process. A similar position has been espoused by Lawrence Hedges (1992) in his book, *Interpreting the*

Countertransference: "the transference-countertransference dimension affords an opportunity for experience with and interpretation of various forms of *personal relatedness styles* and concerns" (p. 200, italics ours). Hedges suggests that one way of analyzing relatedness styles is through developmental metaphors which he classifies into age and theme-related categories: (1) focused attention versus affective withdrawal (age < 6 months); (2) symbiosis and separation (age < 24 months); (3) rapprochement (age 24–36 months); and (4) triangulation (age 36+ months). Hedges identifies transference and countertransference themes associated with each developmental metaphor. He states,

> empathic resonance is taken to mean the analyst's capacity for and willingness to engage in a personal relatedness experience with the person who comes for analysis…countertransference responsiveness may be viewed as closely related to empathy and the interpretive process. (p. 200)

In summary, this brief historical overview of empathy in psychodynamic approaches to treatment reveals that the concept has a central role in psychotherapy. In reviews of the literature (e.g., Hedges, 1992; Maroda, 1991; Pearlman & Saakvitne, 1995; Slakter, 1987; Tansey & Burke, 1989; Wolstein, 1988) there is uniformity in the opinion that empathy is (1) an ability and process related to therapeutic interpretations; (2) associated with the analysis of the meaning of transference and countertransference; (3) a style of interpersonal relatedness; (4) different from the constructs of counteridentification and projective identification; and (5) manifest in degrees of "higher and lower" forms relative to the adequacy of "doing the work" of accurately maintaining empathic attunement to the patient's inner psychological process (i.e., internal working models or schemas of experience). These areas of consensus are useful, since they identify missing operational definitions of these constructs. For example, are the "relatedness styles" suggested by Hedges (1992) measurable? If so, what defines different styles of relatedness? How are styles of relatedness associated with higher and lower forms of empathy? What constitutes higher empathy? If we were to carefully examine a videotaped chronology of psychotherapy with a consensually agreed-upon expert clinician possessing "high empathic skills" of the type noted by Kohut as efficacious, what actions, affects and relatedness styles would distinguish this clinician from someone with "low empathic skills"? If counteridentification processes and "affect signals" are importantly associated with the internal cognitive processing of therapeutic interactions, to what extent could a therapist objectively or subjectively report those *internal* events in a manner that could be correlated to the external, discernible aspects of high degrees of empathy? These questions are not only heuristically important, but they are also directly relevant to understanding the role of empathy in the treatment of psychological trauma and PTSD.

EMPATHIC ATTUNEMENT VERSUS EMPATHIC SEPARATION

In moving towards a theoretical and empirically operational definition of "high empathy," as suggested by Kohut (1982), we start by defining empathic attunement and empathic strain.

First, let us review the continuum of empathic functioning. As a dynamic, variable process, empathic attunement ranges from minimal to optimal, with interval points on this continuum. The continuum of empathic functioning is also associated with the continuum of Type I (avoidance) and Type II (overidentification) countertransference processes which have discernible and measurable subtypes. Moreover, empathic attunement is characterized by six *qualitative dimensions* which are critically important when defining "high" versus "low" empathic functioning. These qualitative dimensions are similar to those identified by Daniel Stern (1985) in his research on infant–mother interactional sequences, and include (1) resonance; (2) intensity; (3) timing; (4) accuracy; (5) prediction; and (6) over-all isochronicity in responding. It is important to differentiate these dimensions of empathy because they identify both *functions* and *processes* in the phenomena of empathic responding which are listed in Figure 5.1.

- **Resonance**
  Function: To accomplish signal communications between dyad members
  Process: Performing phasic synchronization of communication

- **Intensity**
  Function: To achieve affect modulation of physiological/psychological arousal
  Process: Governing control over signal intensity

- **Accuracy**
  Function: To ensure precision of signal decoding, knowing or inferring data
  Process: Accurately tracking signal transmissions

- **Prediction**
  Function: To anticipate future behavioral patterns based on processed data
  Process: Generating informative data about interaction sequence

- **Isochronicity**
  Function: To establish hierarchy of empathic response sequence
  Process: Maintaining "flow" in patterns of synchrony and timing

- **Timing**
  Function: To sustain steady flow of information
  Process: Securing appropriate time response sequences

Figure 5.1 Functional and process dimensions associated with qualities of empathy. Copyright John P. Wilson, 2003.

QUALITY OF EMPATHIC ATTUNEMENT IN POST-TRAUMATIC TREATMENT

The six qualitative dimensions of empathic attunement permit a more detailed analysis of empathic processes in post-traumatic treatment and other forms of psychotherapy. While these dimensions are interrelated, they are also separate processes with their own unique characteristics. For example, if there were optimal attunement, we would expect to see consistently good resonance, proper and flexible affect modulation associated with decoding signal transmissions, combined with transference and verbal reports of the patient's internal working model of psychological states, memories and cognitive schemas. A steady flow of data would be generated which allows the therapist to anticipate and predict behavioral patterns because of good isochronicity and response matching over time. In other words, isochronicity (empathic matching, congruence, phasic synchrony) establishes a *hierarchical algorithm* in the therapist's cognitive understanding of dyadic interactions. This hierarchical algorithm is encoded data of the patient's motivational dynamics, the data being stocked in cognitive "storage files." It is, in essence, an integrated cognitive schema which establishes the nature of past behavioral patterns and interactional styles across a variety of situational contexts, and enables informed, predictive hypotheses about the client's future behavior.

QUALITIES OF EMPATHIC ATTUNEMENT AND CORE EMPATHIC CAPACITIES

The qualitative dimensions of empathic attunement are also related in important ways to the dimensions of empathy, as summarized in Figure 4.4 (see chapter 4). We review these four dimensions here:

- *Empathic Capacity*—the magnitude and limits in maintaining attunement
- *Empathic Resistance*—the scope and capability of the response system to resist being overloaded by stressor demands
- *Empathic Tolerance/Sensitivity*—the extent of system tolerance and the precision of empathic congruence in dyadic interaction
- *Empathic Endurance*—the degree of perseverance and stamina available to sustain empathic attunement

As noted earlier, these core empathic capacities are assumed to be a function of genetic dispositions, developmental socialization, ego-maturity, life experiences and the therapist's trauma history (Eisenberg et al., 1997; Ickes, 1997; Staub, 1979). It is our observation that the core dimensions of empathy have a strong causal relationship to the qualities of empathic attunement which may develop through clinical training, education and experience.

Figure 5.2 summarizes the dynamic interrelationship between the psychological factors comprising the *infrastructure of empathic attunements* in their various forms of manifestation. By analyzing the nature of this relationship, we can now specify in greater detail "higher versus lower" forms of empathy during the course of post-traumatic therapies. The quality and functional capacities of empathy are thought to exist on a continuum, from lower to higher forms of empathic functioning.

HIGHER VERSUS LOWER FORMS OF EMPATHY

The identification of the core dimensions of empathy (i.e., capacity, resistance, tolerance/sensitivity, endurance) and their specific qualities (resonance, intensity, timing, accuracy, prediction, isochronicity), together with their operationalizable criteria as to *process* and *function*, allows for the analysis of high versus low empathic functioning.

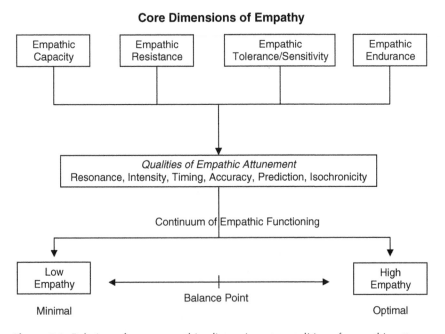

Figure 5.2 Relation of core empathic dimensions to qualities of empathic attunement. Copyright John P. Wilson, 2003.

High Empathy	Low Empathy

Personal Attributes of Therapist

• Optimal Attunement	• Minimal Attunement
• Accurate Empathy (identification)	• Inaccurate Identification
• Accurate Tracking of Client's Internal States	• Inconsistent Tracking of Client's Internal States
• Accurate Signal Detection	• Poor Signal Detection
• Accurate Signal Decoding	• Poor Signal Decoding
• B-Cognition (Maslow)	• D-Cognition (Maslow)
• Altruistic	• Egoistic
• Isochronicity, Phasic Synchrony, Flow	• Dyschronicity, Asynchronous, Blockage
• Congruent Responding	• Incongruent Responding
• Resonant, Harmonic	• Discordant, Inharmonic
• Minimal Distortion	• High Distortion, Noise
• Focally Receptive	• Minimally Receptive
• High Connectivity	• Low Connectivity
• Phasic Continuity	• Phasic Discontinuity
• High Affect Modulation	• Low Affect Modulation
• Good Timing Cadence	• Poor Timing Cadence
• High Empathic Tolerance/Sensitivity	• Low Empathic Tolerance/Sensitivity
• High Empathic Endurance	• Low Empathic Endurance
• High Empathic Resistance	• Low Empathic Resistance
• High Empathic Capacity	• Low Empathic Capacity
• Meta-Cognition of Others	• D-Cognition of Others
• Generativity in Perception and Responsiveness	• Self-limited/Contained
• Sense of Immediate Presence	• Distancing
• Meta-Dissociative	• Dissociative

Figure 5.3 Higher versus lower forms of empathy. Copyright John P. Wilson, 2003.

High Empathic Functioning as the Basis of Optimal Therapeutic Effectiveness

High empathy reflects the ability to be optimally attuned to the client. The high empathy therapist has the competence to understand internal psychological processes accurately, to read emotional states precisely, and to maintain a focal receptive attitude "uncluttered" by signal distortions or contaminated by personal needs. The high empathy therapist is able to identify with the client as if the latter were himself; in other words, he *empathically transposes* himself into the psychic state of being the patient, entering the reality of the patient's world of experience as if it were the therapist's own. The high empathy therapist also has the capacity to use any of the five PTSD symptom clusters (Wilson, Friedman, & Lindy, 2001) as portals of entry into the client's ego-space and interior vault of the unconscious. Understanding the five PTSD clusters enables accurate signal detection and the "decoding" of information being transmitted through the primary channels: affect, defense, somatic states, ego-states, personality processes, unconscious memory (i.e., dynamic repressed), implicit memory and cognitive and perceptual modalities (Wilson, Friedman, & Lindy, 2001).

The high empathy therapist manifests B-cognition (Maslow, 1968, 1970) and has a superior capacity to perceive the client holistically in terms of organismic functioning. Such therapists have a *meta-cognitive* ability to relate in altruistic ways to others, seeing them "as they are at the moment" without a need to change or alter the percept of the trauma client's injuries, impairments or potentially permanent scars to the body, personality or spirit.

High empathy therapists maintain focal receptivity through phasic continuity and connection with the trauma client's flow of emotions, thoughts and fluctuating ego-states, including ego-defenses. They have an "immediate sense of presence" which is experienced by trauma clients as comfort, security and awareness that the therapist is attuned to their needs in a reassuring way. This helps the patients relax, calm down, feel safe and experience less emotional arousal, vulnerability and uncertainty. High empathy therapists have a good cadence in their communicative response sequence. The cadence is measured by accurate signal reception, tracking and decoding of the patient's internal working model of the psychological processes. It is flexibly responsive to the client. As a consequence of accurate empathy (i.e., tracking, signal detection and decoding), the high empathy therapist experiences meta-dissociative states of suspended attention and focal perceptive processes in which they have resonance, groundedness, and effortless "flow" with the stream of associations emanating from the client. This meta-dissociative state is possible, in part, by having high levels of empathic capacity, affect modulation, endurance and stress tolerance which enables empathic processes to operate at their highest potential.

High empathy persons manifest *generativity in attitudinal disposition*. Their attitudinal focal receptivity of the client is concerned with recovery and healing in order to restore normal functioning and self-actualizing potentialities. However, this "attitudinal generativity" is not necessarily age-related in an Eriksonian sense (Erikson, 1968), although it is probably more evident in mature and "well-seasoned" therapists. In high empathy persons, the altruistic, generative attitude is an expression of higher forms of human relatedness which transcend setting, culture, time and space. High levels of empathy are allostatically positive and saluto-genic in nature (see chapter 11 for a discussion). In a metaphorical sense, high empathy persons experience the inner reality of others as if seen through God's eyes.

Characteristics of Low Empathic Functioning

Low empathic functioning is characterized by minimal empathic attunement to the inner psychological state of others. Low empathy therapists lack the ability to understand the trauma client's internal working model accurately. These therapists do not have sufficient empathic capacity, endurance, sensitivity or resistance to sustain empathic resonance consistently. Their focal responsiveness is inconsistent in nature and manifests phasic discontinuity with the "ebb and flow" of the trauma client's dysregulated affective states.

Low empathy therapists' difficulty in modulating affect disrupts their capacity for signal detection, signal decoding and accurate identification with the client's internal state. As a consequence of insufficient affect modulation, *phasic discontinuity* exists in dyadic interactions (see chapter 11). The therapist's receptive capacity is unable to remain "tuned" to incoming signals in the seven channels of transmission, and "drifts off" frequency reception and amplitude modalities, resulting in noise, distortion and interference.

Low empathy therapists manifest deficiency-based cognition (D-cognition; Maslow, 1968, 1970). Their perceptions of the trauma client are strongly influenced by their deficiency-based needs (D-needs) for safety, love, belongingness and esteem (Maslow, 1970; Pearlman & Saakvitne, 1995). The predominance of D-cognition limits the ability of these therapists to perceive the trauma client holistically and accurately. However, low empathy therapists are aware of their heightened level of affect arousal when working with trauma clients, and seek to reduce tension, inner states of anxiety, apprehensiveness and uncertainty. As therapists, they use defenses, including the rigid maintenance of a "blank screen" façade, to mask their inner distress, insecurity, uncertainty or feelings of incompetence, inadequacy or frustration at lacking the knowledge or ability as to how to respond in a different and more efficacious manner.

The low empathy therapist lacks a sense of the "here and now" dynamics during treatment. This absence of connectedness becomes apparent in different ways: clinical coldness; detachment; indifference; and lack of a transparent, deeper understanding of the client's traumatized state of being. The client's perception of such nonconnected detachment or attitudinal insouciance results in the need for guardedness in the face of uncertainty about the therapist's competence. This mistrust and wariness are due to phasic dysynchrony and variable cadence in the communication-response sequence. The client senses that the therapist's tracking of their internal states is inadequate and not "on target," and fails to generate good affective resonance. The client's preconscious and "third ear" tells him/her that something is not "quite right" and automatically evokes defenses.

The low empathy trauma therapist does not manifest meta-dissociative states which would allow fuller empathic congruence. The therapist is self-contained and self-limiting, and this state inevitably results in affective distancing. The trauma client's distress strikes the most vulnerable personality dimension of the therapist. This process occurs quickly and outside of conscious awareness (Knox, 2003). Nevertheless, it activates ego-defensive processes to deal with disturbed emotional reactions, setting in motion a cascade of effects which significantly attenuates the therapist's empathic capacity, sensitivity, endurance, and stress tolerance capacity.

RELATIONAL BALANCE BETWEEN MODES OF EMAPTHIC ATTUNEMENT AND EMPATHIC STRAIN

In the treatment of psychological trauma and PTSD, there exists a transference-countertransference balance beam which is depicted in Figure 5.4.

The modes of empathic attunement and empathic strain are counter-forces in post-traumatic treatments of PTSD and associated conditions of co-morbidity. Clinical work with traumatized patients involves a dysregulating of affect, generated by the power of the patient's trauma story. Dalenberg (2000) has stated: "the intensity of the traumatic transference,

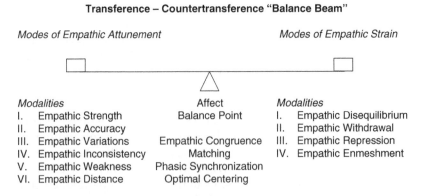

Figure 5.4 Relational balance between modes of empathic attunement and empathic strain. Copyright John P. Wilson, 2002.

and thus, in many cases, the traumatic countertransference, can over-whelm both participants" (p. 14). This potential to experience affective dysregulation poses a risk factor to sustaining empathic attunement, since empathic strains can develop into complete countertransference processes. As Figure 5.4 illustrates, the inherent problem in intense dyadic interaction is to maintain a balance point which permits empathic con-gruence and phasic synchronization with the trauma client's internal psy-chological states. Hence the problem of maintaining a level balance beam during the course of post-traumatic therapy. To understand this problem in greater depth, it is necessary to examine the different modalities of empathic attunement and empathic strain.

DIMENSIONS OF EMPATHIC FUNCTIONING: A CONTINUUM OF ATTUNEMENT TO SEPARATION AND DETACHMENT

Empathic functioning exists on a continuum which ranges from minimal to optimal functioning in terms of empathic attunement. The continuum represents *qualities* of empathic functioning at any given time in the course of post-traumatic therapy. The specific quality or adequacy of empathic attunement spans the spectrum, from none (absent or disen-gaged) to partial to optimal connection and active engagement with the patient. A conceptualization of the continuum of empathic attunement is dynamic in nature and mirrors the reality that many factors influence the *disposition* to empathic functioning (detachment vs. attunement), ranging from clinical experience in trauma work, personal history, fatigue and stress-related states to the raw power of the patient's trauma story to evoke strong affective reactions and countertransference processes in treatment.

EMPATHIC ATTUNEMENT: HIGH EMPATHY AND VIRTUAL ENGAGEMENT

The continuum of empathic functioning is a useful means to consider the adequacy of active therapeutic engagement with the patient. Minimal empathic functioning—the absence or partial achievement of empathic attunement signifies the therapist's failure to relate to the client in a manner that manifests therapeutic congruency. In contrast, therapeutic empathic congruency implies that the therapist, by virtue of his knowledge of the trauma client's internal ego-state, *understands* the trauma experience, even if the client cannot verbalize all of their inner thoughts, feelings and memories. In this regard, the therapist "decodes" the flow of information emanating from the trauma client, and "receives" it without distorting "noises," "signals" or defenses generated by the attempt to match understanding (i.e., congruent empathy) of the client's trauma experience.

The "matching" process of adequate "signal" detection and responsive communication includes both "here and now" processes and the traversing back in time into the subjective reality of the patient's trauma experience. In that regard, it is as if the therapist enters the patient's memory in virtual reality and rides along like a fellow passenger on a journey of discovery in which the patient says: "Look at this experience, this event or situation, and see what happened here long ago." Together, much like two persons taking a ride in an adventure park, they *experience* memories and emotions in a common flow which reveals the nidus of the trauma experience. In sharing the reliving of the trauma together, the therapist exerts much energy and concentration to attune empathically to the client while, at the same time, maintaining "third eye" observation and protection of interpersonal boundaries.

Clearly, this is among the reasons that led Kohut (1977) to consider empathy as a process of knowing or data collection. However, to be an accurate recorder or "collector," the trauma patient's data requires four interrelated dimensions of empathic functioning: (1) empathic capacity; (2) empathic tolerance and sensitivity; (3) empathic endurance; and (4) empathic resistance. It is important to recognize that the strains imposed on the process of attunement in post-traumatic therapy may cause empathic breaks or ruptures. A rupture, cessation or sudden loss of empathic attunement reflects the inability to continuously track, understand and accurately experience another person's ego-states and frame of reference (Wilson & Lindy, 1994). Understanding the factors that lead to a disruption in empathic functioning is necessary for identification of the traps, pitfalls, and potential trouble areas imposed by compassion fatigue, burnout, vicarious traumatization, overwhelming affective responses and the existence of disruptive countertransference (Figley, 2002; Pearlman & Saatvikne, 1995; Wilson & Lindy, 1994).

STRUCTURAL DIMENSIONS OF EMPATHIC FUNCTIONING

The basic dispositions in empathy of movement towards attunement with, or separation from, the client allows us to specify more precisely the four interrelated dimensions of empathic functioning: (1) capacity, (2) resistance, (3) tolerance and sensitivity, and (4) endurance. Each of the primary dimensions has two basic subcomponents (i.e., conceptual axis and features) which further define the process by which functioning on a *continuum* of empathic attunement can be understood and empirically observed *in vivo*, during treatment or in experimental research (Ickes, 1997; Wilson, Friedman, & Lindy, 2001; Wilson & Lindy, 1994).

Empathic Capacity: Structural Dimension I

In the most fundamental sense, empathic capacity refers to the magnitude of capacity available to maintain empathic attunement. The determinants of variations in individual capacity include genetic factors (e.g., temperament), personality characteristics (e.g., self-esteem, locus of control, fortitude, level of moral development, ego-strength and mature vs. immature ego-defenses), experience of working with trauma clients, and "clinical load" demands (i.e., the quantum and frequency of work with trauma patients).

Empathic Resistance: Structural Dimension II

Empathic resistance refers to the forces that impose strains on the process of empathic congruence, matching or attunement. Strains and distress during the treatment tax empathic ability and, if not managed properly, lead to powerful affective reactions, countertransference processes or inadequacy in functioning in an optimal way with empathic congruence. In an earlier work, we detailed the categories or determinant classes of empathic strains and countertransference which include (1) the intensity and power of the trauma story; (2) personal factors of the therapist; (3) specific factors concerning the patient (e.g., gender, age, type of trauma, personality style, etc.); and (4) institutional and organizational factors which adversely impact a positive therapeutic stance with the trauma patient (Wilson & Lindy, 1994).

The recognition of the sources, "triggers," and idiosyncratic manifestations of empathic strains and therapists' "resistance operations" as defensive security measures is critical for the successful outcome of post-traumatic therapy. In our earlier research (Wilson & Lindy, 1994), we discussed four modes of empathic strain which included: (1) empathic disequilibrium, (2) empathic enmeshment, (3) empathic repression, and (4) empathic withdrawal which were associated with Type I (avoidance) and Type II (overidentification) countertransference styles.

Empathic Tolerance & Sensitivity: Structural Dimension III

Empathic tolerance is related to empathic capacity, in the sense that tolerance refers to the ability to endure both transference and TST. It is the aptitude to bind personal affective reactions generated in response to the trauma story, to control the affective intensity of a treatment session or to effectively modulate personal emotions aroused by the process.

Empathic sensitivity denotes the *precision* of "signal detection," "decoding," empathic congruency; the capacity to control tension; and the ability to effectively use personal affective reactions (i.e., inform knowledge about the therapeutic process) and cognitive images, fantasies, perceptions, memories and thoughts to maintain empathic attunement efficiently. Further, empathic sensitivity necessarily involves accurate and detailed "decoding" of transference projections. Thus, the greater the empathic sensitivity, the greater the "match" in self-object understanding. MacIsaac and Rowe (1991), referring to Kohut's work, state: "the primary function of empathy was to make possible the painstaking unfolding of a patient's inner experiences and the emergence of specific developmental needs (self-object transferences)" (p. 21). Thus, empathic tolerance and sensitivity are dual interrelated processes in the continuum of empathic disposition.

Empathic Endurance: Structural Dimension IV

Empathic endurance connotes the degree of perseverance and capacity to sustain the ongoing process of empathic attunement. Empathic endurance reflects the volume and quality of psychological energy available to engage in the attunement process, to find ways to creatively use the portals of entry into the ego-space and inner sanctum of psychological functioning, especially the complicated intrapsychic elements of identity and self (Wilson, Friedman, & Lindy, 2001). The capacity for endurance, combined with tolerance and sensitivity, is directly associated with the therapist's psychological well-being.

MODES OF EMPATHIC ATTUNEMENT

Understanding the continuum of empathic attunement as a spectrum of possible behavioral dispositions, ranging from detachment to empathic congruence, response matching and connection with the trauma patient, we can now further define six modes of empathic attunement. As will be discussed later, these six modes interact dynamically with the four primary modes of empathic strain (disequilibrium, enmeshment, repression and withdrawal) to create the structure and process of affective responses and countertransference in the treatment of PTSD. These six modes of empathic attunement are not discrete, "concrete" modalities of behavioral orientation. Rather, they are dynamic processes that represent degrees of empathic attunement. However, as Figure 5.5 illustrates, each modality has its own set of characteristics which define the quality of the interactional sequence during the treatment process, and can be observed and assessed in vivo or by questionnaires (Dalenberg, 2000; Wilson & Thomas, 1999).

I. **Empathic Strength**

   (a) *Defining Conceptual Axis*: Attunement – Endurance

   (b) *Features*: Empathic strength, affective equilibrium and containment, perseverance, stamina, openness to experience, cognitive complexity, divergent thinking, mature ego-defenses, phasic synchronization

II. **Empathic Insufficiency**

   (a) *Defining Conceptual Axis*: Attunement – Separation

   (b) *Features*: Empathic insufficiency, low perseverance, affective guarding (closed), immature ego-defenses, emotionally detached, potentially exploitative

III. **Empathic Weakness**

   (a) *Defining Conceptual Axis*: Resistance – Separation

   (b) *Features*: Empathic weakness, insufficiency, unresponsiveness, withdrawal, denial, repression of personal affect, defensive controls, ineffective responses, immature ego-defenses, easily overwhelmed with anxiety

IV. **Empathic Inconsistency**

   (a) *Defining Conceptual Axis*: Attunement – Resistance

   (b) *Features*: Empathic inconsistency, variability in: attunement, matching congruence; disequilibrium, counterphobic, potential enmeshment, fluctuating affect modulation (overcontrol-undercontrol of emotional arousal)

V. **Empathic Accuracy**

   (a) *Defining Conceptual Axis:* Attunement – Sensitivity/Tolerance

   (b) *Features*: Empathic accuracy, precision in matching, congruency, affect modulation, mature ego-defenses, naturalness and authenticity in responding, cognitive complexity, phasic synchronization

VI. **Empathic Distancing**

   (a) *Defining Conceptual Axis*: Separation – Sensitivity/Tolerance

   (b) *Features*: Empathic distance, isolation, avoidant inadequacy, counterphobic, low affect modulation, insufficient matching, phasic desynchronization

---

Figure 5.5 Modes of empathic attunement. Copyright John P. Wilson, 2002.

Empathic Strength: EA Mode I

Defining Conceptual Axis: Attunement—Endurance

Figures 5.6 and 5.7 present a summary of the six modes of empathic attunement. These six dimensions are process variables, and define discrete subtypes of empathic attunement. As such, they reflect behavioral propensities at any given time in dyadic interaction.

Empathic strength is a mode of empathy in which attunement exists, being in phasic sequence or flow with the patient, and establishing response congruency to transference dynamics. Empathic strength also connotes the therapist's stamina, perseverance, and endurance in

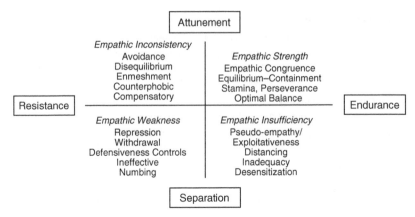

Figure 5.6 Modes of empathic attunement. Copyright John P. Wilson and Jacob D. Lindy, 2002.

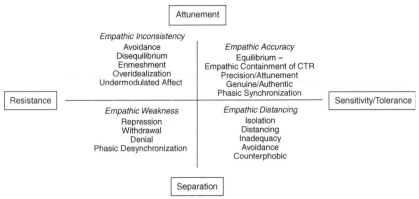

Figure 5.7 Modes of empathic attunement. Copyright John P. Wilson and Jacob D. Lindy, 2002.

maintaining a grounded (i.e., equilibrium) containment of the patients and their own affective responses.

Empathic Insufficiency: EA Mode II

Defining Conceptual Axis: Attunement—Separation (Detachment)
Empathic insufficiency is a mode of responding in which a deficiency is evident during the therapeutic interaction, due, in part, to the disposition

towards separation and detachment. The many expressions or forms of empathic insufficiency include (1) inability to contain self and patient affect; (2) loss of connection with "phasic" communication in the transference; (3) loss of attention, concentration and focus, resulting in an empathic break; (4) inadequacy in timing, intensity or resonance; and (5) exploitativeness. Pseudo-empathy is a form of empathic insufficiency which may lead to conscious or unconscious exploitation of the patient for personal, narcissistic gratification. Wolstein (1988) has characterized this pattern as aggressive-dependent and states,

> An aggressive-dependent analyst is remarkably different because he will respond to his patient in a direct and straightforward manner…because his own desire for dependency and warmth has not been satisfied, he will falter in his direct, straightforward attitude with his patient when they touch on basic questions of intimacy and warmth. Out of conditions of his own past, he will lose his firm grip of the patient's problem and experiences, and he will act out in an obstructive manner, hindering the relationship just because he is anxious and frightened by his patient's requirements. (p. 229)

Thus, empathic insufficiency, in any of its vicissitudes, will result in some degree of ineffectiveness in sustaining empathy with the trauma client.

Empathic Weakness: EA Mode III

Defining Conceptual Axis: Resistance—Separation
Empathic weakness reflects a fundamental inability to connect, get in phasic synchronicity with the patient and respond with matching congruence. Empathic weakness is associated with an overly guarded, anxious and self-contained therapist who is unlikely to manifest, or self-disclose, affect in facial channels (i.e., "blank façade," therapeutic mask). Such therapists are prone to withdrawal, repression and defensive avoidance of engaging the more difficult of the patient's experiences in trauma. As a defensive measure, they may rigidly rely on a technique of treatment (e.g., EMDR, CBT) as avoidance of attunement with the patient's "here and now" dynamics. Reliance on a structured method of treatment removes the need for authentic experiential encounters with the trauma patient—thus providing an illusion of safety, and reinforcement of belief in the efficacy of the technique.

Empathic Inconsistency: EA Mode IV

Defining Conceptual Axis: Attunement—Resistance
Empathic inconsistency is characterized by fluctuations in the quality and precision of attunement capacity. Empathic inconsistency is associated

with states of disequilibrium, tendencies towards compensatory enmeshments and boundary crossings or, alternatively, counterphobic maneuvers and tactics and defensive operations. However, what makes the mode of empathic inconsistency different from the mode of empathic weakness is that the therapist is disposed towards attunement with, rather than separation from, the client. Empathic inconsistency is especially evident in inexperienced trauma therapists and those with a personal history of trauma (Wilson & Thomas, in press).

Empathic Accuracy: EA Mode V

Defining Conceptual Axis: Attunement—Sensitivity/Tolerance
Empathic accuracy is the metaphoric "twin sibling" of empathic strength. Empathic accuracy is characterized by precision in matching capacity for affect modulation, naturalness and authenticity in responding, and cognitive complexity (see Davis & Kraus, 1997, for a review of personality variables and empathy). Empathic accuracy, when combined with empathic strength, makes for optimal attunement in treatment. *Therapists with empathic accuracy and strength will demonstrate the highest levels of quality in interaction*: (1) resonance (tuning, phasic sync, flow); (2) intensity (matching congruency over time); (3) timing (maximally effective timing of responsiveness); (4) accuracy (precision of signal detections, decoding and translation); and (5) prediction (the cognitive skill to predict, anticipate or foresee future behavioral reenactments that are trauma-based, or that reflect the patient's characterological dynamics).

Empathic Distancing: EA Mode VI

Defining Conceptual Axis: Separation—Sensitivity/Tolerance
Empathic distancing is characterized by separation, affect, and overcontrol of responsiveness by the therapist who attempts to maintain a controlled emotional distance from the patient. The therapist engages in isolation, counterphobic behaviors, insufficient matching (incongruence), and displays a low capacity to effectively regulate affect. There is a pronounced tendency to maintain a blank façade persona as a defense against inner uncertainty, vulnerability and insecurity.

MODES OF EMPATHIC STRAIN: THERAPISTS' REACTIVE STYLES

The experience of empathic strain occurs when empathic attunement gets challenged, overwhelmed or rendered inadequate in the face of the patient's transference or self-presentation, as part of the dyadic or group interactional sequence. Empathic strain may be experienced in a variety of ways that can result in completely countertransferential processes. However, empathic strain is typically manifest as increased tension, anxiety, problems of "focus" in concentration or attention, or increased autonomic nervous system activity (heart rate, respiration, etc.). Empathic strain may also appear in somatic forms as muscle tension, sleepiness or drowsiness, gastric distress, headaches, fatigue, or more idiosyncratic reactions such as rubbing ones eyes, localized muscle spasms and urinary urgency. Further, empathic strain may be conscious or unconscious in nature, and potentially associated with rapid shifts in emotional states (e.g., anger, disdain, fear, horror) and cognitive processes (e.g., fantasies of escape, rescue, thoughts about nonclinical activity, etc.).

Empathic strain results from those interpersonal events in psychotherapy that weaken, injure or force, beyond reasonable limits, a positive

---

I. **Empathic Disequilibrium**

   (a) *Defining Conceptual Axis*: Normative, objective affective reactions and disposition to Type II–countertransference (normative–over-identification) associated with reactions to trauma story

   (b) *Features*: Empathic strain, experienced disequilibrium of personal states; shifts in well-being, uncertainty, vulnerability and security

II. **Empathic Withdrawal**

   (a) *Defining Conceptual Axis*: Normative, objective affective reaction and disposition to Type I countertransference (Normative–Avoidance) associated with personal reactions to trauma story

   (b) *Features*: Withdrawal from empathic attunement, separation, avoidance and security operations (i.e., unconscious defense processes), feelings of uncertainty and inadequacy; reliance on blank façade, misperceptions of transference

III. **Empathic Enmeshment**

   (a) *Defining Conceptual Axis*: Personalized idiosyncratic reactions to trauma story and disposition to Type II (overidentification) countertransference

   (b) *Features*: Personalized affective reactions; activation of personal issues; tendency to cross boundaries; overinvolvement with patient; excessive amplification of attunement responses; reciprocal dependency

IV. **Empathic Repression**

   (a) *Defining Conceptual Axis*: Personalized idiosyncratic reactions to trauma story and disposition to Type I (avoidance) countertransference

   (b) *Features*: Personal repression of memories, conflicts and unresolved problems aroused by interactional sequence with patient. Loss of attunement may be severe and damaging to therapeutic outcome. Withdrawal, denial and distancing are all defensive operations

---

Figure 5.8 Modes of empathic strain. Copyright John P. Wilson, 2002.

therapeutic response to the client. Countertransference processes are only one source of empathic strain, yet we believe that in the treatment of PTSD, CTRs are perhaps the primary cause of treatment failure.

Building on the seminal works of Cohen (1952), Figley (1995, 2002), Hedges (1992), Wolstein (1988), Tansey and Burke (1989), Slatker (1987), Danieli (1988), Lindy (1987), Dalenberg (2000), Wilson (1989), Maroda (1991), Wilson and Lindy (1994) and Ickes (1997), it is possible to construct a schema for understanding modalities of empathic strain in the treatment of PTSD. Figure 5.9 illustrates these forms of empathic strain in a two-dimensional representation, based on Type I and Type II modes of CTRs, crossed by the axis of objective and subjective countertransference processes. Objective CTRs are expectable, affective and cognitive reactions experienced by the therapist in response to the client's personality, behavior and trauma story. Subjective CTRs are personal reactions which originate from the therapist's own personal conflicts, idiosyncrasies or unresolved issues from life-course development.

Type I and Type II modes of countertransference refer respectively to the primary tendencies of counterphobic avoidance, distancing and detachment reactions, as opposed to tendencies to overidentify and become enmeshed with the client. Type I CTRs typically include forms of denial, minimization, distortion, counterphobic reactions, avoidance, detachment and withdrawal from an empathic stance towards the client. Type II CTRs, in contrast, involve forms of overidentification, overidealization, enmeshment and excessive advocacy for the client, as well as behaviors that are elicited by guilt reactions.

As Figure 5.9 illustrates, the combination of the two axes of countertransference processes produces four distinct modes or styles of empathic strain, which we have identified as (1) *empathic withdrawal*, (2) *empathic repression*, (3) *empathic enmeshment* and (4) *empathic disequilibrium*. Although a therapist may experience one style or reaction pattern more than another, it is possible to experience any or all of the modes of empathic strain during the course of treatment of a traumatized client (see Wilson & Lindy, 1994, for an extended discussion).

THE FOUR MODES OF EMPATHIC STRAIN

Empathic Withdrawal: ES Mode I

Defining Conceptual Axis: Normative Reactions and Type I CTR
Empathic withdrawal is a mode of countertransference strain which occurs when the therapist experiences expected affective and cognitive reactions during treatment, and he or she is predisposed, by defensive style and personality characteristics, towards Type I avoidance and detachment responses. In this mode, a rupture occurs in the empathic stance towards

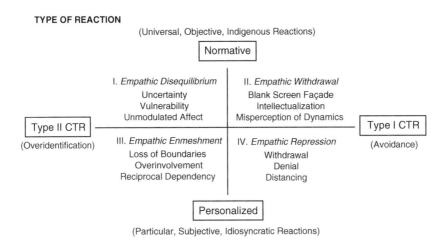

TYPE OF REACTION

(Universal, Objective, Indigenous Reactions)

Normative

I. *Empathic Disequilibrium*
Uncertainty
Vulnerability
Unmodulated Affect

II. *Empathic Withdrawal*
Blank Screen Façade
Intellectualization
Misperception of Dynamics

Type II CTR
(Overidentification)

Type I CTR
(Avoidance)

III. *Empathic Enmeshment*
Loss of Boundaries
Overinvolvement
Reciprocal Dependency

IV. *Empathic Repression*
Withdrawal
Denial
Distancing

Personalized

(Particular, Subjective, Idiosyncratic Reactions)

Figure 5.9 Reactive style of therapist. Copyright John P. Wilson and Jacob D. Lindy, 1994.

the client. The result is often the loss of capacity for sustained empathic inquiry, due to overreliance on the "blank screen" or conventional, or recently delegated or taught (for the new therapist), therapeutic techniques. These reactions block the painful task of integrating the trauma experience, and may lead the therapist to misperceive or misinterpret the behavior and psychodynamics of the client, on the basis of previous assumptions.

Empathic Repression: ES Mode II

Defining Conceptual Axis: Personal Reaction and Type I CTR
A similar process occurs in *empathic repression,* in which the transference issues of the patient reactivate conflicts and unresolved personal concerns in the therapist's life. Thus, a personalized subjective reaction, combined with a disposition towards a Type I CTR, may be associated with repressive countermeasures by the therapist. His or her inward focus on areas of personal conflict is likely to be associated with an unwitting and unconscious withdrawal from the therapeutic role, and denial of the full significance of the clinical issues being presented by the client.

Empathic Enmeshment: ES Mode III

Defining Conceptual Axis: Personal Reaction and Type II CTR
The third mode of strain, *empathic enmeshment,* is the result of the therapist's tendency toward Type II CTRs, coupled with subjective reactions

during treatment. In this mode of empathic strain, the clinician leaves the therapeutic role by becoming overinvolved and overidentified with the client. The most common consequences are pathological enmeshment and a loss of role boundaries in the context of treatment. In the treatment of PTSD, therapists with a personal history of trauma and victimization are especially vulnerable to this mode of empathic strain, and may unconsciously attempt to rescue traumatized clients as an indirect way of dealing with their own unintegrated personal conflicts (Wilson & Thomas, 2000). Perhaps the greatest danger that occurs within this mode of empathic strain is the potential for the therapist to unconsciously reenact personal problems through pathological enmeshment. When this occurs, it not only causes an abandonment of the empathic stance towards the person seeking help, but may also lead to secondary victimization or the intensification of transference themes that the patient brought to treatment in the first place.

Empathic Disequilibrium: ES Mode IV

Defining Conceptual Axis: Normative Reaction and Type II CTR
Empathic disequilibrium, as Figure 5.9 indicates, is characterized by a disposition to Type II CTRs and the experience of objective reactions during treatment, especially in work with patients suffering from PTSD and co-morbid conditions. This mode of strain for the therapist is characterized by somatic discomfort, feelings of insecurity and uncertainty as to how to deal with the client, and more. It occurs commonly in therapists who experience either Type I or Type II CTRs.

It is interesting to note that one consequence of empathy is that the therapist may experience degrees of hyperarousal that are proportional to the level of hyperarousal the patient manifests as part of the PTSD. Clearly, this is a type of dual unfolding in the dynamics of transference and countertransference. It is another example of parallelism in empathic congruence and matching phenomena.

TRANSFORMATIVE PROCESSES BETWEEN MODES OF EMPATHIC ATTUNEMENT AND EMPATHIC STRAIN

The relationship between modalities of empathic attunement and empathic strain is like that of two participants on a balance beam, each anchoring one end while trying to stay balanced with the fulcrum point of the flat board between them. Empathic attunement is a dispositional orientation, and empathic strain is an inevitable, indigenous process in post-traumatic therapies. Modes of empathic attunement and strain are dual processes which may occur simultaneously in concert with each other or, alternatively, progress in a slowly evolving sequence until the strain becomes manifest, conscious and observable.

Figure 5.10 presents an overly simplified but heuristically useful way of illustrating the relationships among modes of empathic strain and empathic attunement. The figure depicts the primary and secondary relationships between the six modes of empathic attunement and the four modes of empathic strain. It also indicates which countertransference type (I or II) is associated with each relationship. For example, both empathic strength and empathic accuracy are primarily associated with empathic disequilibrium and, secondarily, with empathic enmeshment tendencies, and both are Type II countertransference styles (overidentification). On the other hand, empathic insufficiency, inconsistency and weakness are strongly associated with primary relationships of empathic withdrawal or repression, Type I countertransference patterns (avoidance, detachment). Interestingly, all three of these modalities are also prone to empathic enmeshment and problems in maintaining proper, effective therapeutic

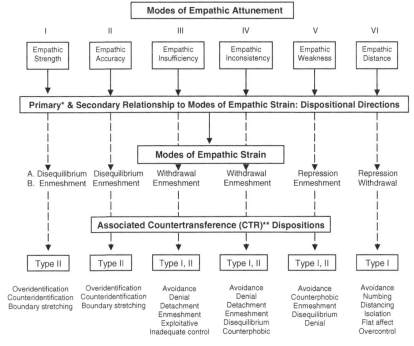

Figure 5.10 Transformative processes between modes of empathic attunement and empathic strain. Copyright John P. Wilson, 2002.

boundaries, and may therefore vacillate between Type I and Type II CTR styles. Finally, we can also see that empathic distancing is related to modes of empathic strain, characterized by Type I (avoidance) countertransference in the primary form of withdrawal and repression.

It is important to recognize that the relationships described are dynamic processes and reflect predominant patterns of modal interactional sequences in the treatment process. Clearly, there are many possible combinations of possibilities, depending on the factors that influence the process (e.g., the quality of attunement, empathic capacity, the power of TST to overcome coping and defenses, etc.).

EMPATHIC ATTUNEMENT AND AFFECT REGULATION IN THE THERAPEUTIC DYAD

Among the keys to maintaining empathic attunement in post-traumatic therapy is the management of affect by the therapist which, in turn, directly impacts the manner in which the patient perceives and experiences the therapeutic alliance. Empathic attunement and states of high empathy are characterized by synchrony in the therapeutic dyad which includes states of matched physiological synchrony.

In a review of laboratory studies of physiological synchrony and empathic accuracy based on studies of marital couples, menstrual cycles in university female roommates, heart rate synchrony between mothers and neonates, heart rate changes of clients and their therapists, Levenson and Ruef (1997) stated,

> ...physiological *synchrony* is also clearly *intertwined* with processes of emotional synchrony, especially those of emotional support and emotional knowledge. This closeness of connection is underscored by the evidence of *bi-directionality causality*—emotional synchrony can produce physiological synchrony, and physiological synchrony can produce emotional synchrony. (p. 68–69, italics ours)

This research evidence is especially relevant to clinical work with PTSD, since trauma patients not only experience intense affects (e.g., anger, rage, grief), but such intense emotional states are also chronically dysregulated as part of the psychobiological substrate of PTSD (Friedman, 2000a, 2002b, 2004; Schore, 2000). Thus, the reciprocal and bi-directional influence necessary in post-traumatic therapy involves strong, dysregulated affects being transmitted by the patient (sender) in the seven channels to the therapist (receiver). At the same time, these affects create stressor demands with a high probability of causing dysregulated affects (i.e., empathic strains). Thus, the central problem of the balance beam is the arduous process of maintaining *affect balance* between modes of empathic attunement and empathic strain. Empathic attunement is physiological and emotional synchrony; empathic strain is affect dysregulation— physiological and emotional dysynchrony of the bi-directional type studied by Levenson and Reuf (1997).

In understanding the psychobiology of empathy, transference and countertransference in post-traumatic therapy, the role of dysregulated affects in both the patient *and* the therapist is critical. Traditionally, focus in clinical settings on countertransference has been on therapist reactions. However, as experimental research informs us, this is insufficient for a fuller analysis and view of the dynamics that occur in the therapeutic dyad. Moreover, Allan Schore (2003) has noted, in his comprehensive integrative synthesis of the literature, *Affect Regulation and the Repair of the Self,* dysregulated affective states in the patient are *transmitted through therapeutic attachments, that is, transferential relationship modes with the analyst*:

> *In order to receive these transferential communications of traumatically dissociated affect,* the therapist must shift from a left to right hemispheric dominant state of evenly hovering attention…an *empathic state* in which, according to Kohut, "the deeper layers of the analyst's psyche are open to the stimuli which emanate from the patient's communication while the intellectual activities of the higher levels of cognition are temporarily largely selectively suspended." (p. 143, italics ours)

Schore's (2003) research strongly suggests that it is parsimonious to consider self-pathologies (including PTSD and trauma-related personality disorders) as *"deficits of affect regulation* that result from an arrest of emotional development" (p. 279, italics ours). In his statement of principles of psychotherapeutic treatment of self-pathologies, Schore states that empathic attunement and the management of dysregulated emotional states is important:

> an understanding of therapeutic empathy, a major mechanism of the treatment, as not so much of a match of left brain verbal cognition but as a right brain nonverbal psychobiological *attunement, and the use of affect, synchronizing transactions for interactively generating and amplifying positive affect that forges the patient's attachment to the therapist.* …An understanding that the *therapist's affect tolerance is a critical factor* determining the ranges, types, and intensities of emotions that are explored or disavowed in the transference-countertransference relationship and the therapeutic alliance. (p. 281, italics ours)

Schore (2003) is suggesting that the synchronization of affects (i.e., isochronicity) facilitates the generation of positive emotional states in client *and* therapist. This perceived sense of positive affective in the ther-

apeutic dyad enhances attachment processes. We suggest that the generation of a positive emotional climate in post-traumatic therapy increases
the quality of TST processes in terms of their structural dimensions: (1)
content imagery of trauma story; (2) complexity/intensity of trauma
experience; (3) ambiguity/clarity of transference projections; (4) TST
themes; and (5) affect arousal potential (AAP).

In the context of a positive-affective therapeutic milieu, the trauma
patient will disclose more clearly and completely the specific nature of the
trauma experience. Further, with the client's attachment to the therapist
strengthened, as also to empathic attunement, trust, comfort level, the
perception of a safe sanctuary for disclosure and containment of affects,
etc., the trauma patient will be able to tolerate processing the horrific and
overwhelming aspects of the trauma experiences. Stated differently, with
the *reduction of anxiety* (i.e., affect dysregulation) in *both* therapist and
patient (i.e., decreased hyperarousal associated with reexperiencing
trauma), it will be easier to cognitively process and bring perspective to
the traumatic experience and how it relates to life-course development. In
a similar perspective, Schore (2003) suggests that, in terms of the dynamic
interaction processes occurring during treatment,

> a moment-to-moment tracking of content-associated subtle and dramatic
> *shifts in arousal and state in patient narratives*, and the identification of non-
> conscious "hot" cognition that trigger nonlinear discontinuities of right
> brain and therefore *dysregulate self-function*. (p. 280, italics ours)

This passage is particularly insightful since it underscores the fact that
PTSD patients often manifest, moment to moment, "subtle and dramatic
shifts in arousal" and psychological states which include dissociation,
altered (nondissociative) ego-states, affect-driven hyperarousal conditions and disposition to high risk acting-out behaviors (Wilson, 1989,
2004; Wilson, Friedman, & Lindy, 2001; Wilson & Zigelbaum, 1986).
However, with the presence of good empathic attunement, the PTSD
therapist can monitor more precisely the fluctuations in affect "moment
to moment" and "treatment session to treatment session" throughout the
course of therapy. As noted earlier, empathic attunement is characterized
by six dimensions: (1) resonance; (2) intensity; (3) accuracy; (4) prediction; (5) timing; and (6) isochronicity. All these six dimensions are
involved in monitoring and tracking the patient's trauma transference
transmissions during treatment. Thus, affect balance in the therapist is as
important to the successful outcome of post-traumatic treatments as is
the capacity of the PTSD or trauma patient to faithfully report their
symptoms and the pathogenic effects of psychological functioning, self-
processes, ego-identity and overall sense of well-being as a person.
As Schore (2003, p. 283) indicates, *poor affect tolerance* will likewise be a

critical factor in determining the "range, types, and intensities of emotions that are … [avowed] or disavowed in the transference–countertransference relationship…" In our view, then, this is the dilemma of the balance beam—the creation of a positive emotional environment for treatment in which there is a solid therapeutic alliance, positive affective attachment by the patient, a genuine sense of safety, security and trust which optimally facilitates the process of post-traumatic therapy.

To summarize, Figure 5.11 illustrates the factors influencing critical affect tolerance by the therapist in post-traumatic therapies. As noted in chapter 4, the core determinants of empathic disposition include (1) genetics, (2) socialization, (3) ego-maturity and moral development, (4) trauma history, and (5) life experiences. These factors are correlated with high and low empathic dispositions whose characteristics were presented

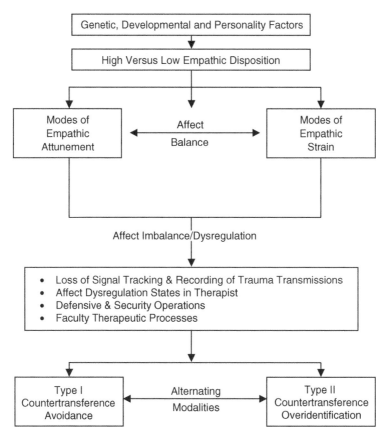

Figure 5.11 Factors influencing critical affect tolerance by therapist in post-traumatic therapy. Copyright John P. Wilson, 2003.

in Figure 4.3. Empathic dispositions, together with training, education and experience, influence the therapist's capacity to maintain empathic attunement or experience counterproductive and disruptive empathic strains. When *affect intolerance* or *imbalance* occurs in the therapist, it leads to (1) a loss of signal tracking and decoding of trauma transmissions; (2) state of affect dysregulation; (3) defensive and security states; and (4) faulty therapeutic processes. The results of this set of interacting processes are forms of Type I and Type II CTRs, which themselves function in alternating modalities and subtypes. When this state of CTR alteration occurs, the balance beam begins to tilt, and the therapist's task is to find the fulcrum which restores balance and equilibrium.

REFERENCES

Bennett, M. (2001). *The empathic healer: An endangered species.* New York: Academic Press.

Cohen, M. B. (1952). Countertransference and anxiety. *Psychiatry, 15,* 231–243.

Dalenberg, C. (2000). *Countertransference and PTSD.* Washington, DC: American Psychological Association Press.

Dalenberg, C. L. (2000). *Countertransference in the treatment of trauma.* Washington, DC: American Psychological Association Press.

Danieli, Y. (1988). Confronting the unimaginable: Psychotherapists' reactions to victims of the Nazi Holocaust. In J. P. Wilson, Z. Harel, & B. Kahana (Eds.), *Human adaptation to extreme stress* (pp. 219–237). New York: Plenum Press.

Davis, M. H. & Kraus, L. A. (1997). Personality and empathic accuracy. In W. Ickes (Ed.), *Empathic accuracy.* New York: Guilford Publications.

Eisenberg, N., Murphy, B. C. & Shepard, S. (1997). Developmental aspects of empathic accuracy. In W. Ickes (Ed.), *Empathic accuracy* (pp. 73–117). New York: Guilford Publications.

Erikson, E. H. (1968). *Identity, youth and crisis.* New York: Norton.

Figley, C. R. (1995). *Compassion fatigue.* New York: Brunner/Mazel.

Figley, C. R. (2002). *Treating compassion fatigue.* New York: Brunner-Routledge.

Friedman, M. J. (2000a). *Posttraumatic and acute stress disorders.* Kansas City, MO: Compact Clinicals.

Friedman, M. J. (2000b). *Post-traumatic stress disorder: The latest assessment and treatment strategies.* Kansas City, MO: Compact Clinicals.

Friedman, M. J. (2004). Psychobiology and pharmacological approaches to treatment. In J. P. Wilson, M. J. Friedman & J. D. Lindy (Eds.), *Treating psychological trauma and PTSD* (pp. 94–125). New York: Guilford Publications.

Hedges, L. (1992). *Interpreting the countertransference.* Northvale, NJ: Jason Aronson.

Ickes, W. (1997). *Empathic accuracy.* New York: Guilford Publications.

Knox, J. (2003). *Archetype, attachment, analysis.* London: Brunner-Routledge.

Kohut, H. (1977). *The restoration of the self.* New York: International Universities Press.

Kohut, H. (1982). Introspection, empathy and the semi-circle of mental health. *International Journal of Psychoanalysis, 63,* 395–407.

Levenson, R. W. & Ruef, A. M. (1997). Psychological aspects of emotional knowledge. In W. Ickes (Ed.), *Emapathic accuracy* (pp. 44–73). New York: Guilford Publications.

Lindy, J. D. (1987). *Vietnam: A casebook.* New York: Brunner/Mazel.

MacIsaac, J. & Rowe, T. S. (1991). *Empathic attunement.* New York: Analytic Press.

Maroda, K. J. (1991). *The power of countertransference.* New York: Wiley.

Maslow, A. H. (1968). *Towards a psychology of being.* New York: Van Nostrand.

Maslow, A. H. (1970). *Motivation and personality.* New York: Harper.

Pearlman, L. & Saakvitne, K. (1995). *Trauma and the therapist.* New York: Norton.

Schore, A. N. (2000). Attachment and regulation of the right brain. *Attachment & Human Development, 2,* 23–47.

Schore, A. N. (2003). *Affect regulation and the repair of the self.* New York: Norton.

Slakter, E. (1987). *Countertransference.* Northvale, NJ: Jason Aronson.

Staub, E. (1979). *Positive social behavior and morality.* New York: Academic Press.

Stern, D. (1985). *The interpersonal world of the infant.* New York: Basic Books.

Tansey, M. J. & Burke, W. F. (1989). *Understanding countertransference.* Hillsdale, NJ: Erlbaum.

Wilson, J. P. (1989). *Trauma, transformation and healing: An integrated approach to theory, research and post-traumatic theory.* New York: Brunner/Mazel.

Wilson, J. P. (2004). PTSD and complex PTSD: Symptoms, syndromes and diagnoses. In J. P. Wilson & T. M. Keane (Eds.), *Assessing psychological trauma and PTSD* (2nd ed., pp. 1–47). New York: Guilford Publications.

Wilson, J. P., Friedman, M. J. & Lindy, J. D. (2001). *Treating psychological trauma and PTSD.* New York: Guilford Publications.

Wilson, J. P., Harel, Z. & Kahana, B. (1989). The Day of Infamy: The legacy of Pearl Harbor. In J. P. Wilson (Ed.), *Trauma, transformation and healing: An integrated approach to theory, research and post-traumatic theory* (pp. 129–159). New York: Brunner/Mazel.

Wilson, J. & Lindy, J. (1994). *Countertransference in the treatment of PTSD.* New York: Guilford Publications.

Wilson, J. P. & Thomas, R. (1999). *Empathic strain and counter-transference in the treatment of PTSD.* Paper presented at the 14th annual meeting of the International Society for Traumatic Stress Studies, Miami, FL.

Wilson, J. P. & Thomas, R. (in press). Issues in the diagnosis and understanding of compassion fatigue, secondary traumatic stress and vicarious traumatization. *International Journal of Emergency Mental Health.*

Wilson, J. P. & Zigelbaum, S. D. (1986). PTSD and the disposition to criminal behavior. In C. R. Figley (Ed.), *Trauma and its wake* (Vol. 2, pp. 305–321). New York: Brunner/Mazel.

Wolstein, B. (1988). *Essential paper on countertransference.* New York: New York University Press.

6

Empathic Rupture and Affect Dysregulation: Countertransference in the Treatment of PTSD

In the treatment of PTSD and its associated co-morbidities, empathic attunement and psychobiological synchrony mean that the therapist is "in phase" with the client. To be "in phase" and synchronized with a patient can refer to various psychological and physiological phenomena, especially in work with trauma clients. Experimental research has examined the phenomenon of therapists' reactions to their patients and found evidence for response matching of autonomic nervous system functioning. Levenson and Ruef (1997) state,

> With the exception of those times when the therapist was said to be distracted by other concerns, they found that heart rate changes during these episodes were generally similar for both patient and therapist ... the *thera-pist's and patient's heart rate moved in similar directions as the levels of tension varied, but moved in opposite directions when the patient showed antagonism toward the therapist.* (p. 48, italics ours)

Consistent with our views on the role and significance of empathy in PTSD treatment, in particular, and trauma work more generally (i.e., emergency medicine, disaster response, acute intervention, critical incident debriefing), Levenson and Ruef (1997) suggest that empathic accuracy involves a parallelism between two individuals in a variety of contexts, including psychotherapy: "... empathic accuracy—a state in which one person (the subject) can accurately tell what another person (the target) is feeling—will be marked by *psychological parallelism* between the subject and target" (p. 62).

Psychological parallelism can be thought of as part of the core mechanisms that govern empathic attunement, matching phenomenon and response congruence in the treatment of trauma clients. However, this is precisely where the potential difficulty lies, because research evidence has found that affective intensity (e.g., therapist exposure to the power of trauma stories and ultimate horror; hostility towards the therapist; etc.) is associated with "distraction" or a loss of empathic attunement. The receiver's capacity to sustain precise signal decoding is disrupted due to internal emotional states (e.g., fear, anxiety, uncertainty), and simultaneously activates dysynchronous defensive-security operations to quell the disrupted state of equilibrium or to reduce tension (empathic strain) created by the loss of synchrony (see chapter 10 for a further discussion). Levenson and Ruef (1997) suggest a similar formulation from experimental research and state: *"that high physiological arousal on the part of the sender is associated with low accuracy in the receivers' ratings of the targets' affect"* (p. 61, italics ours). This finding has direct relevance and application to the treatment of PTSD, since traumatic events constitute the extreme end of the continuum of stressful life events. Beyond doubt, the patient's reports of life-threatening, horrific, dangerous or catastrophic experiences have the potential to induce *maximum affective arousal* in the therapist.

The voices and faces of trauma patients confront therapists on a regular basis with emotionally laden, disturbing and often shameful accounts of human encounters with fragmenting effects of trauma. Abyss experiences of trauma present the therapists with reports of encounters with the darkest episodes of human existence, and the specter of injury or death at the hands of fate or calculated, willful human malevolence (Wilson, 2003). To sustain empathy effectively, the therapist must open the self to the uncomfortable parallelism of the patient's dysregulated affect, pain, and struggle to overcome the injuries. Empathic strains, strong affective reactions and countertransference reactions (CTRs) are indigenous to PTSD treatment. The question is: how are they best managed in the service of maintaining empathic attunement to the inner reality of the patient's experiences? And further, what happens if there is a rupture of empathy?

IMPACT OF EMPATHIC STRAIN AND COUNTERTRANSFERENCE ON THE PSYCHOTHERAPY OF TRAUMA SURVIVORS

The understanding of empathic stress permits analysis of the factors that determine CTRs and how CTRs, in turn, affect the phases of stress recovery, and potentially cause pathological results for the client. What happens to the treatment process and the phases of recovery when there is a loss of empathic attunement? What ensues when there is a loss of physiological and psychological synchrony? What are the causes of anxiety and defensiveness in the therapist?

Many sources of empathic strain in the treatment of trauma patients can result in complex countertransference processes (Wilson & Lindy, 1994). As summarized in Figure 6.4, four primary factors influence the manifestation of CTR during the treatment process: (1) the nature of the trauma story and the description of intense traumatic experiences involving death, injury, dying, exposure to the grotesque, horror, catastrophic disaster, chaos, etc.; (2) the therapists' personal characteristics, including their trauma history, personality style, defensive structure, capacity for affect modulation, and high vs. low empathy disposition; (3) institutional/organizational factors (e.g., adequacy of resources, client population); and (4) specific demographic and characterological features of the client's trauma experience, etc. Each of these four categories of CTR determinants reflects the reality that powerful affective reactions can be provoked in therapists, throwing them off balance and necessitating a grim struggle to maintain empathic attunement.

Consider the following case vignette. It is a true account of a torture victim, for whose therapist one of us (JPW) was asked to provide supervision in an underfunded mental health agency in a large metropolitan city of over five million people.

CASE EXAMPLE: TERESA'S ABYSS OF NO RETURN

Teresa Sanchez (alias), a woman in her early 20s, had been accepted for treatment at a state-sponsored community mental agency which assists asylum seekers, refugees and torture victims. After necessary preliminaries, Teresa told her therapist the following trauma story of her internment in a South American prison for political dissenters. Disturbed by what the client disclosed, the therapist requested an immediate consultation (JPW). Moreover, it should be noted that neither was Teresa a political activist nor was she involved with the government in any capacity. She was a single mother of two young girls, Maria and Julia, aged 5 and 8, respectively, and an ordinary citizen residing in her hometown of Malaqueña.

Teresa was raped and sexually tortured by her captors. She was also subjected to sensory deprivation: electrodes were attached to her nipples and clitoris while she was "spread-eagled" on the bare floor of her unsanitary, roach-infested 6' × 9' cell. Her captors laughed at her while they tortured her with electric-powered generators and then demeaned her by urinating on her body, calling her a worthless "bitch" and "whore." Later, after repeated torture sessions, they unleashed specially conditioned German Shepherd dogs who snarled and growled at her, then bit her breast, drawing blood. Next, the well-trained dogs had sexual intercourse with her, while her captors watched, laughed and made humiliating remarks: "Look at you—you fuck dogs—you are a real bitch, you slut of a whore."

After being "hooded" (sensory deprivation), Teresa was subjected to mock executions: her captors would "lock and load" AK-47 automatic rifles next to her head, and expose her to the sounds of gunshots and screams of actual executions and beatings. After months of repeated torture in various depraved forms, Teresa was forced to watch as her captors beheaded her two young girls. They then kicked the severed, bleeding heads, with vacant wide open eyes, as "soccer balls." Teresa was finally returned to her cell and forced to eat food on the floor "like a dog." After nine months of imprisonment she was released, and she sought asylum as a refugee in a foreign country outside of South America.

At the time she was received at the mental health center, Teresa was living alone on public welfare. She was suffering from suicidal ideation, major depression, traumatic bereavement and PTSD. She expressed doubts whether counseling would help her, and could communicate only in broken English.

The therapist, Annette, who was assigned to Teresa's case, was about the same age, engaged to be married and wanted to start a family. Annette identified with her client's gender, role status, age and emotional predicament. She identified with Teresa as a woman who had been raped, tormented and repeatedly abused by her male captors. As one who had specialized in working with asylum seekers, Annette was keenly aware of Teresa's struggle to start life over again in a new country, without a family, job, friends or any tangible emotional anchors. Initially overwhelmed by Teresa's story, she feared that Teresa would commit suicide. Despite her years of experience in working with asylum seekers, Annette was also racked by uncertainty and doubt about whether or not she could help the depressed, suicidal torture victim. She even considered referring her elsewhere for treatment. However, there was no other treatment center for Teresa, and Annette knew that, despite her fears and uncertainty, the responsibility for Teresa's care would ultimately rest with her alone. Annette confided that she hoped that her years of dedicated service would give her the coping skills to help Teresa whose life was complicated by the secondary stresses of relocation, poverty, unemployment, asylum seeking and overcoming of traumatization. She also confided that she sensed that "more was yet to come," that what she had heard was only part of Teresa's trauma story.

The case history of Teresa Sanchez, which has been presented many times at conferences and educational courses, always stirs powerful affect in those who hear it. No one has ever reported being unaffected by listening to this case vignette, though men and women react differently to the trauma story. Men's thoughts turn aggressive, and their fantasies center around retaliation against the captors. Women respond like Annette, identifying with Teresa as a woman, mother, and victim of intrusive male aggression.

When members of the audience are asked to describe their personal reactions to Teresa's story, the responses cover the entire spectrum of emotional, somatic and cognitive possibilities. For example, many participants report somatic complaints such as stomach upset, a lump in the throat, nausea, faintness, muscle tension, head or heart pounding, clenched fists and holding of breath. Emotional responses include feelings of fear, dread, apprehension, anger, rage and sadness. There is a wide range of cognitive reactions: disbelief that this is a true case history; disavowal of the existence of such torture; denial that this could happen; dissociative-like states, including an altered sense of presence in the conference room, inattention and mentally drifting. Other cognitive-affective reactions include anger directed towards me for "telling the story," a wish that I had not told the story or had stopped before Teresa was raped by the dogs and her children executed.

A few professionals report overintellectualization. For example, in presenting Teresa's story at a conference in Europe on one occasion, I was approached by a psychiatrist who narrated to me the history of beheadings, and the use of severed heads in political domination and the mockery of victims dating from the 9th century A.D. What I found curious in his overintellectualized reaction was the "matter of fact way" in which he related to the horror of Teresa's story as also to the gruesome history of beheadings. I wondered what he would have done, in a professional role, if Teresa had been his patient. For example, would he have told her the history of beheading and its use as political power? Would he have intellectually minimized the emotional trauma of watching her only children mercilessly hacked to death?

PSYCHOBIOLOGICAL MECHANISMS OF COUNTERTRANSFERENCE: DUAL UNFOLDING PROCESSES IN CLIENT AND THERAPIST

We can now extend our analysis of the role of empathic attunement and empathic strain to an understanding of the psychobiology of countertransference in the treatment of trauma and PTSD. In an oversimplistic sense, countertransference processes reflect the tilting of the balance beam discussed in chapter 5. When empathic strains, caused by *dysregulated affective processes in the therapist*, become excessive and inadequately modulated, they run the risk of becoming full-blown CTRs. It should be noted that this is a naturally occurring process which varies in degree among therapists.

Different types of CTRs get enacted during the course of treatment. First are the readily identifiable Type I and Type II CTRs in the treatment of trauma victims and PTSD (Wilson & Lindy, 1994). Then there are also *compensatory CTRs* of various sorts, especially when a therapist realizes the extent and nonfunctionality of a particular type of CTR. Further, specific ego-defenses are associated with different types of empathic strains, compassion fatigue, vicarious traumatization and countertransference

(Dalenberg, 2000; Danieli, 1988; Figley, 1995, 2002; Pearlman & Saatvitne, 1995; Tansey & Burke, 1989; Wilson & Lindy, 1994). Nevertheless, despite the nature and type of countertransference, there exists a common psychobiological pathway which underpins these reactive mechanisms. At the center of these processes is the issue of *dysregulated affects* and their internal processing by the therapist during the "moment to moment tracking of content-associated subtle and dramatic shifts in arousal and state in patient narrations" (Schore, 2003a, p. 280).

Figure 6.1 illustrates the common psychological pathways in empathic strains and countertransference processes. To chart the operation of the "twin," simultaneous processes of affect and psychological states in countertransference, the diagram artificially separates the dual unfolding processes that occur in the transference-countertransference matrix. The patient discusses the trauma related experiences while the therapist

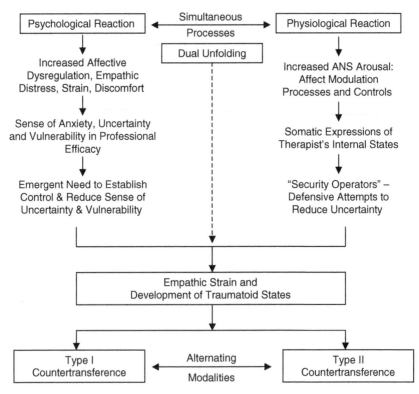

Figure 6.1 Therapists' reactions to trauma clients: Affect dysregulation and dual unfolding processes. Copyright John P. Wilson, 2003; John P. Wilson and Jacob D. Lindy, 1994.

listens, experiences affective reactions, analyzes both the internal working model of the client's frame of reference and the therapist's own internal processes stirred by the patient's narrative. Hence, these are two sets of unfolding processes, described originally by Henry Racker (1968) as "dual unfolding processes."

Let us try to understand the nature of the dual unfolding process in more detail. First, in terms of psychological reactions, the therapist experiences varying levels of affect, empathic strain and empathic attunement. When empathic strain becomes significant, it gives rise to a sense of anxiety, uncertainty or confusion about professional efficacy or the "right course of action." The experience of anxiety may then lead to the need to establish control and predictability in relation to ongoing transactions. The experienced, internal need to reduce anxiety may be conscious or unconscious. It is typically associated with the need to reduce uncertainty and feelings of vulnerability. The greater the degree of affect dysregulation stirred by the patient's trauma narrative, the greater the need to defend against it and to find ways to bind anxiety and modulate the levels of anxiety, fear, uncertainty or sadness. This, then, results in the nidus of empathic strains which, in turn, generate forms of countertransference.

Second, the *psychological reactions* which co-occur in the dual unfolding process include increased autonomic nervous system (ANS) arousal associated with dysregulated affective states. These affective states range on a continuum from micro-disturbances to overwhelmingly powerful, irrepressible displays of empathic distress. Moreover, as inner states of anxiety are experienced, they are accompanied by *somatic expressions of internal states* which include the following: flushing; increased heart rate and respiration; sweating; neck aches and headaches; motor agitation and shifting body positions; stomach upset; a lump in the throat; increased parastolic activity; blank facial expressions; nervous smiling; stammered or pressured speech patterns; increased or decreased voice volume; and nervous gestures and gaze avoidance. These manifestations of internal states are then followed by "security operations" in which the therapist attempts to reduce uncertainty, feelings of vulnerability and dysregulated affects. These "security operations" are directly correlated with countertransference processes of Type I (avoidant, counterphobic, detached) or Type II (overidentification, enmeshment, rescuer, prosocial advocacy, etc.).

DIMENSIONS OF TYPE I AND TYPE II COUNTERTRANSFERENCE

Type I and Type II CTRs fall along a continuum of therapeutic relationship styles (Hedges, 1992). In post-traumatic therapies, both Type I and Type II CTRs are experienced during treatment. As will be discussed in chapter 9, there are different forms of Type I and Type II CTRs, and practitioners usually manifest a predominant modality (e.g., Type II, overidentification, excessive advocacy), with subtypes of behavioral reactions reflecting the operation of defenses, compensatory actions or interactive dynamics with a client.

In Type I CTRs, empathic strains, generated by compassion fatigue, vicarious traumatization and dysregulated affect, cause the therapist to leave the stance of empathic attunement and "move away" from the client. As noted by Wilson and Lindy (1994),

> What activates the various forms of avoidant CTRs is a set of psychobiological processes which are experienced either consciously or unconsciously as an uncomfortable sense of uncertainty, anxiety, and insecurity in terms of how to best help the person suffering from PTSD and associated symptoms. (p. 42)

Thus, in Type I avoidant forms of CTR, the therapist moves away from empathic attunement at multiple levels: cognitive, perceptual, intellectual, affective and interpersonal.

THE CONTINUUM OF TYPE I AND TYPE II COUNTERTRANSFERENCE

Figure 6.2 presents a summary of the continuum of Type I countertransference processes and six categories of subtypes which range from denial of PTSD as a diagnosis, or as perceptual denial and failure to see the patient's PTSD symptoms in context, to more active forms of disengagement. In the Type I withdrawal subtype, for example, the therapist may simply refer the clients to another agency or diagnose them as "poor candidates" for treatment, due to "Axis II" personality disorder factors. Similarly, another form of withdrawal from active therapeutic engagement, in which the detailed trauma history is explored in depth, is to prescribe medication for symptom reduction. While pharmacotherapy is quite useful in the treatment of PTSD (Friedman, 2001), it requires relatively little of the doctor's time. It does not require the painstaking task of gradually discovering the full and complete chronology of the patient's trauma history.

The continuum of Type I avoidant CTRs (denial minimization, distraction, avoidance, detachment and withdrawal) represents degrees of avoidance and detachment from the therapeutic alliance. The Type I avoidant CTRs range from the subtle and unconscious to the obvious and willful in nature. Further, Type I CTRs reflect a loss of empathic attunement and are the product of empathic strain as a cumulative psychobiological process, as illustrated in Figure 6.1.

Type I and Type II CTRs vary in severity, frequency, duration and periodicity, depending on the interactional dynamics with the patient. For

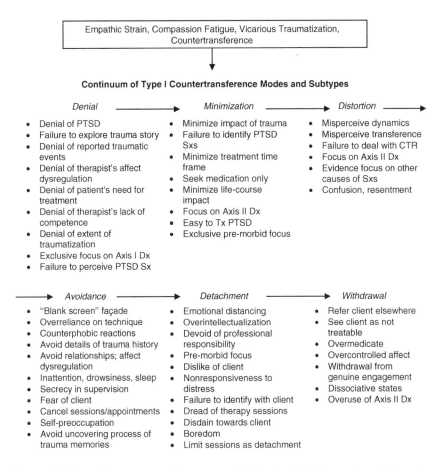

Figure 6.2 Type I countertransference modalities (avoidant, counter-phobic, detachment). Copyright John P. Wilson, 2003; John P. Wilson and Jacob D. Lindy, 1994.

example, in discussing the case example of Teresa (the torture victim), many therapists undergoing Type I CTR express doubts on whether they could tolerate working with the fragility of Teresa's mental state for a long period of time. They express their belief that the intensity of affect experienced in working with Teresa would cause compassion fatigue, vicarious traumatization and simply exhaust their empathic stamina. Would such reactions lead them to cancel appointment sessions or become overly reliant on a "blank screen" façade? Perhaps avoid important details of her trauma story or minimize the time necessary for successful treatment? Or, in an extreme case develop counterphobic rituals during treatment sessions, or drink excessively in the evenings when thoughts of Teresa's story intrude into the serenity of the home?

On the other hand, would the intensity of Teresa's trauma story stimulate strong Type II CTRs or intrapsychic compensatory reactions? Would the reality of Teresa's desperate situation cause the therapist to move back the boundary lines and allow Teresa to telephone the home? Would the therapist become a vocal advocate for the cause of oppressed women who are victims of male-dominated political regimes? Would the therapist feel a special sense of mission to save Teresa from self-destruction, as a waif of a society largely indifferent to her profound suffering and the traumatic bereavement of her children, loss of female sexuality and spiritual wholeness? Would it be a more realistic assessment to suggest that the therapist, treating a patient as difficult as Teresa, would experience a full spectrum of Type I and Type II CTR, alternating subtypes of modalities, as different ego-defenses are utilized by the therapist when empathic strains exceed empathic attunement? From this perspective it can be seen that the

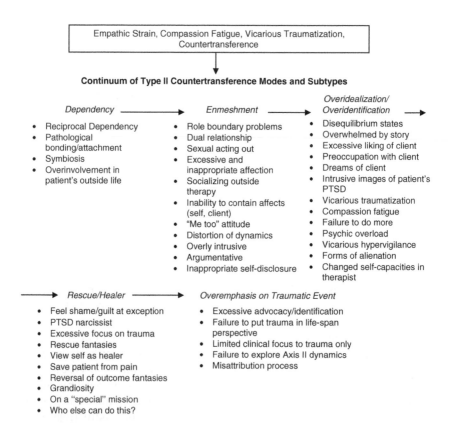

Figure 6.3 Type II countertransference modalities (over-identification, enmeshment, prosocial advocacy). Copyright John P. Wilson, 2003; John P. Wilson and Jacob D. Lindy, 1994.

problem of the balance beam is an ongoing dilemma of maintaining therapeutic equilibrium, not sacrificing professional boundaries and running the risk of being cast into role enactments of various types through trauma transference.

EMPATHIC RUPTURE: COUNTERTRANSFERENCE EFFECTS IN TREATMENT OF TRAUMA AND PTSD

Empathic rupture poses the greatest risk to a therapeutic alliance and the efforts to create a safe holding environment to contain the intense affects associated with traumatization and PTSD. An empathic rupture may take many forms in a therapeutic dyad. They're a degree of severity in empathic break in the therapist's level of phasic synchrony with the patient's trauma transmissions. A rupture of empathy, and loss of a therapeutic role with empathic attunement, can occur at any stage during the treatment process: (1) initiation and uncovering of the trauma history; (2) active processing of the adverse pathogenic effects of trauma; and (3) integration and completion. As a process, either a Type I or Type II CTR can be stimulated by affective dysregulation in the therapist, leading to a loss of empathic attunement. A Type I or Type II CTR modality can emanate from the primary categories which stir CTRs: (1) patient's trauma history; (2) therapist's personality; (3) client's personality; and (4) organizational and institutional factors. These categories of potential determinants of CTRs may individually, jointly or interactively cause an empathic rupture at any chronological point in the time line of psychotherapy and health care treatment. Moreover, once an empathic rupture occurs, it may have either disruptive or pathological damaging effects on the treatment process.

Figure 6.4 illustrates how a rupture in empathy sets up dysregulated affective states in the therapist which lead to CTRs. As a conceptual schema, Figure 6.4 illustrates the "dynamic flow" of empathic strains, countertransference and ruptures in the therapeutic alliance which impact the stress recovery process at any of five phases of post-traumatic treatment: (1) the reexperiencing of trauma; (2) the reconstructed trauma chronology and associated memories; (3) the unfolding of new affect and imagery; (4) reappraisal processes; and (5) assimilation into cognitive schema, integration and completion (Courtois, 1999; Foa, Keane, & Friedman, 2001; van der Kolk, McFarlane, & Weisaeth, 1997; Wilson, Friedman, & Lindy, 2001; Wilson & Lindy, 1994).

POTENTIAL PATHOGENIC OUTCOMES CAUSED BY COUNTERTRANSFERENCE

Figure 6.4 indicates that at least six major categories of potentially pathogenic outcomes are caused by countertransference: (1) cessation or

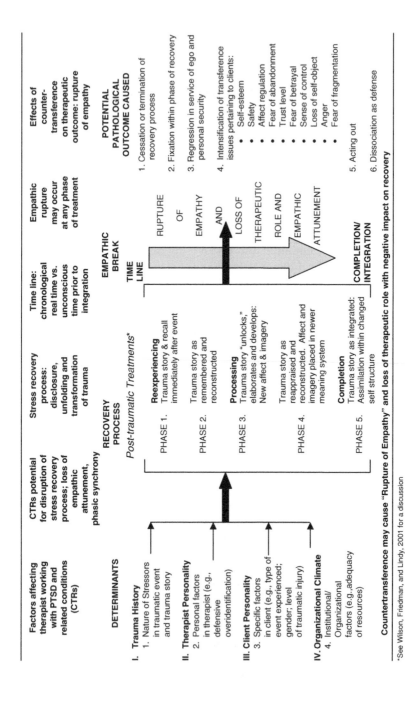

Figure 6.4 Empathic rupture: Countertransference (CTR) effects in the treatment of trauma and PTSD. Copyright John P. Wilson and Jacob D. Lindy, 1994.

premature termination of the recovery process; (2) fixation (stasis) within a phase of stress recovery; (3) intensification of transference issues (e.g., trust, safety, fear of abandonment); (4) acting out behaviors; (5) dissociation; and (6) regression. These six categories represent the most common pathogenic outcomes when a significant rupture of empathy occurs during post-traumatic treatments.

CASE EXAMPLE VIETNAM REDUX: FULL METAL MIND

In considering the range of pathogenic outcomes caused by a rupture in empathy and the loss of empathic attunement, it is useful to highlight another case example. Mike, a highly decorated 18-year old Marine during the Vietnam War, was a patient at his local Veterans Administration (VA) hospital, where a new resident in psychiatry was assigned to him. The young, brash, arrogant resident was the same age as Mike when the latter entered the hospital for treatment after several suicide attempts, binge drinking sagas and dissociative acting out episodes in which he spoke in Vietnamese and stalked his wooded backyard with an AK-47 automatic rifle. The psychiatry resident made a "treatment pact" with Mike that they would talk about his childhood and life after Vietnam, but would refrain from discussing his many combat episodes, including those for which he was awarded the Bronze and Silver Stars for valor as the sole survivor of his Marines Corps platoon which was ambushed by enemy forces in 1968 near An Hoa.

After a week of inpatient treatment, Mike lied to his doctor when he told him that he was feeling well and appreciated being allowed the chance to rest and calm down. The young and woefully inexperienced psychiatry resident granted Mike his first leave pass on a Friday afternoon, instructing him to return after four hours. Mike went binge drinking at a local bar and refused to return to the hospital. He became increasingly suicidal and, in an intoxicated, morose condition, decided to return to his hometown by Greyhound bus. He became agitated, angry and spiteful towards the psychiatry resident whom he found completely unhelpful and cowardly for not wanting to hear all that had happened to him in Vietnam. Mike telephoned a fellow combat veteran who had been a patient in the hospital with him. Through the outreach efforts of a local veteran's group, Mike secured the help of a combat buddy patient and a psychologist with extensive experience with war veterans. The next day Mike returned to the VA hospital. His resident psychiatrist chastised him for acting out and violating his hospital pass privilege. The authoritarian and insecure resident characterized Mike's actions as a "malignant form of regressive acting out." But the truth was that, because of the nature of their "treatment pact," the therapist had not read the patient's file on his Vietnam combat experiences. Had he done so, he might have realized that Mike's violation of his hospital pass occurred on the anniversary of the day his entire platoon had been killed in the August of 1968 while he alone had survived, after single-handedly eliminating 11 enemy soldiers. For this courageous act, he had been awarded a Purple Heart and the "Silver Star" for valor, shortly after turning 18 years of age during combat operations.

When Mike went on a drinking binge during his short hospital furlough, he was reliving his war trauma and other PTSD symptoms, on the anniversary of one of the most terrifying days in his life. After a week of calm, when no further "acting out" problems recurred, Mike was discharged from inpatient treatment by the resident psychiatrist and returned to his rural Ohio hometown. Two days later, he attempted suicide with a .45 caliber pistol which he had brought home from Vietnam and kept in a cedar chest, along with his high school yearbook, his medals from Vietnam, including three Purple Heart awards and photos of his buddies killed in action. Mike never returned for treatment to the VA hospital, but eventually stabilized through the help of Alcoholics Anonymous and a veteran's outreach counseling center.

Mike's case illustrates many of the key pathogenic aspects caused by the loss of empathic attunement and countertransference. Mike ceased going for treatment; fixated in a recovery phase for several years; and experienced dissociative acting out connected with the vivid reliving of traumatic war events on the anniversary of his personal "day of infamy" in 1968 when his closest buddy died in his arms after being shot in the forehead in a paddy field during an ambush by enemy forces. Mike had repressed his emotions, and his PTSD-associated transference issues were intensified by the psychiatry resident's refusal to talk about his combat and war related stressors. Further, it is relevant to our analysis of the pathogenesis caused by the loss of empathic attunement that the young psychiatry resident openly boasted in narcissistic ways about his anti-war protests as a university student, and expounded on why the Vietnam War was wrong and should not have taken place.

To Mike, the young insouciant doctor's anti-war stance and refusal to discuss Mike's own war experiences, which had caused his psychiatric illness of PTSD, suicidal proclivities and depression, were tantamount to betrayal, abandonment and humiliation by an agent (resident psychiatrist) of the U.S. government (the VA Hospital) which had been responsible for sending him to Vietnam. In this sense, Mike experienced a double betrayal, loss of trust and sense of abandonment. He feared that to "open up" would mean self-disintegration and fragmentation. After his suicide attempt following treatment at the VA Hospital, Mike lived alone in secluded isolation for years and drank heavily until a trusted fellow combat veteran took him to meetings of Alcoholics Anonymous. He eventually regained sobriety and, on the anniversary of his last major battle in the Vietnam War, married a woman 17 years younger than himself.

INTENSIFICATION OF TRANSFERENCE DYNAMICS CAUSED BY EMPATHIC RUPTURE

Transference processes, as initially observed by Freud (1917), are ubiquitous in psychotherapy and other helping professions—medicine, crisis debriefing, teaching, counseling, nursing, and so on (Wilson & Lindy, 1994). In the process of transference, a client relates to the therapist in a manner similar to that of his past relationships with other significant associates. Pearlman and Saakvitne (1995) define transference as "the unconscious repetitions in a current relationship of patterns of thoughts, feelings, beliefs, expectations and responses that originated in important early relationships" (p. 100). These two definitions of transference make it apparent that the phenomenon involves reenacting aspects of past relationships in current treatment settings. In post-traumatic therapies, this poweful *reenacting* relationship dynamic is especially important, because the patient establishes a trusting relationship with the therapist who, in turn, may be "cast," "scripted," or "placed" into an unconscious or preconscious set of role relationships with the patient.

More specifically, transference processes are not "all or none" phenomena. They involve the partial manifestations of past emotional hurts and the repetition of previously dysregulated affective states during the traumatic experience. They comprise unconscious reenactments of traumatic situations, events that occurred in the past and partial expressions of encapsulated and dissociated ego-states. Transference processes also involve role-reversal enactments with the therapist, and unconscious nonverbal transmissions of horrifying experiences for which verbal channels of expression are unavailable. They incorporate states of alexythymia (Krystal, 1988) and the operation of thought patterns, belief systems and reinforcement expectancies that functioned in the past and that involved othersin the patient's traumatic event or history. They also include dissociative states as reenactment or symbolic signal transmissions to the therapist in respect of the meaning and structural configuration of symptoms.

TRAUMA TRANSFERENCE AS SIGNAL ENCODED MEMORIES

The 10 transference themes summarized in Figure 6.5 can be considered as TST dispositions to behavioral enactments or reenactments in post-traumatic therapy. These themes are present in the transference as signal encoded memories, usually of an unconscious nature. Themes of TST have their counterparts in CTRs in the various modalities of empathic strain discussed in Chapter 5: empathic disequilibrium; empathic withdrawal; empathic repression; and empathic enmeshment. The dynamics of the various modalities of TST have the power to activate any one of the modalities of countertransference, a fact commented upon by Pearlman and Saakvitne (1995):

> The therapist and client's willingness to notice and name their interpersonal experience allows the *transformative work* with transference and countertransference dynamics in these therapies.... While the provision of an empathic respectful relationship is essential, it is not sufficient to change the deeply entrenched self and object relational paradigms held by survivors of much [sexual] abuse. *A therapist's attunement to her countertransference is an essential tool to her understanding and analyzing the transference.* (p. 119, italics ours)

In post-traumatic therapies, the identification of empathic strains and countertransference, created by the loss of empathic attunement, allows therapists to "work backwards" in the sense that, by understanding the CTRs, they can connect such reactions to the transference dynamics summarized in Figure 6.5.

Stated differently, the trauma specific transference transmissions (TSTT) occur through seven channels of information transmission which originate in the patient's unconscious (i.e., dynamic repressed) and in the patterns of PTSD and co-morbid symptoms. As previously discussed, TSTT are encoded (see Figure 1.1) into affects, defenses, somatic states, ego-states, personality processes, unconscious memories (implicit memories) and cognitive-perceptual phenomena. *These signals contain precise and encoded*

I.	Repetition of previously dysregulated affective states
II.	Manifestations of emotional injuries associated with significant self-objects
III.	Unconscious reenactment of traumatic events, places, persons, situations
IV.	Unconscious reenactment of overwhelming states of fear, helplessness, horror, terror, sadness, etc.
V.	Complete or partial expressions of encapsulated and dissociated ego-states
VI.	Role reversal enactments or reenactments with therapist as abuser, perpetrator, rescuer/savior, parents, co-worker, sibling, etc.
VII.	Unconscious, nonverbal transmissions of unspeakable, horrifying experiences for which verbal channels are unavailable
VIII.	Manifestations of alexythymia and difficulties experiencing and identifying feelings
IX.	Operation of thought patterns, belief systems and reinforcement expectancies that occurred in the past with others involved in the traumatic events or patient's history
X.	Dissociative states as reenactment or as symbolic signal transmissions to therapist as of the meaning and structural configuration of symptoms

Figure 6.5 Universal themes modalities of trauma specific transference and behavioral dispositions in post-traumatic therapy. Copyright John P. Wilson, 2003.

information about the internal working model of the patient's trauma experiences and fluctuating ego-states. Further, these multichanneled sources of information are screened or filtered by defenses which protect the patient's familiar vulnerability. Nevertheless, TSTT contain the critical material for the therapist to decode, analyze and use in treatment. Countertransference processes can impede this therapeutic task. They are also like reciprocal "lock and key" mechanisms, and contain condensed information which is extremely useful in decoding signal transmissions from the patient and gaining resolution relating to the larger constellation of issues to be addressed.

MEANING AND INTERPRETATION OF DUAL UNFOLDING PROCESSES

Figure 6.6 presents a summary of the transference-countertransference matrix of interpersonal dynamics in post-traumatic therapies. The figure indicates the "flow" of interpersonal processes, originating in TSTT (see Figures 1.1 and 1.2) which encode information stored in the implicit and explicit memory in seven separate channels. The seven channels of signal

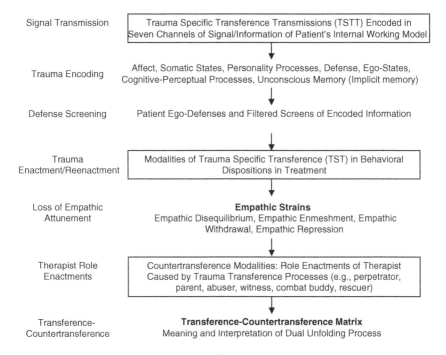

Figure 6.6　The transference–countertransference matrix—Meaning and interpretation of dual unfolding processes. Copyright John P. Wilson, 2003.

transmission (i.e., affects, defenses, somatic states, ego-states, personality processes, cognitive-perceptual processes and unconsciously repressed material) are filtered through defensive screens and then manifest themselves, in projective form, as 10 modalities of TST behavioral dispositions.

The 10 modalities of TST behavioral dispositions are enacted or reenacted during treatment, and influence the onset of empathic strains in the therapist which, in turn, lead to countertransference modalities in the therapist's behavior as responses to TSTT. Finally, this dual unfolding process (Racker, 1968) creates a "matrix" of psychodynamic information which is rich in meaning and critical for analytical interpretation. As Figure 6.6 shows, this complex process originates with the client's signal transmissions from the trauma story and life narrative, and continues through a series of transformative mechanisms which continuously recycle until completion is reached and therapy is complete.

A similar view of this dynamic set of processes has been expressed by Allan Schore (2003b) in his book, *Affect Regulation and the Repair of the Self*, where he refers to Melanie Klein's pioneering work:

> Klein (1946) defined projective identification as a process wherein largely *unconscious information is projected from sender to recipient....* I suggest that if Freud (1912, 1958b) was describing how the unconscious can act as a *"receptive organ,"* Klein's concept of projective identification attempts to model how an unconscious system acts as a *"transmitter"* and how these *transmissions* will then *influence the receptive functions of another unconscious mind.* This clearly implies that the unconscious systems interact with other *unconscious systems, and both receptive and expressive propensities determine their communicative capacities.* (p. 59, italics ours)

What we are suggesting is that not only are there multichanneled dimensions to signal transmissions from patient to therapist which are encoded with information specific to the trauma and life-course experiences, but also that these signals are embedded in transference enactments and reenactments *during* the course of treatments. These signal transmissions occur at all levels of awareness, and contain meanings that are interpretable and are facilitated by empathic attunement and high states of empathic functioning, which we will discuss in greater detail in chapter 11.

REFERENCES

Courtois, C. (1999). *Recollections of sexual abuse: Treatment principles and guidelines.* New York: Norton.

Danieli, Y. (1988). Confronting the unimaginable: Psychotherapists' reactions to victims of the Nazi Holocaust. In J. P. Wilson, Z. Harel, & B. Kahana (Eds.), *Human adaptation to extreme stress* (pp. 219–237). New York: Plenum Press.

Figley, C. R. (1995). *Compassion fatigue*. New York: Brunner/Mazel.

Figley, C. R. (2002). *Treating compassion fatigue*. New York: Brunner-Routledge.

Foa, E., Keane, T. M. & Friedman, M. J. (2001). *Effective treatments for PTSD*. New York: Guilford Publications.

Freud, S. (1917). *Introductory lecture on psychoanalysis*. New York: Norton.

Hedges, L. (1992). *Interpreting the countertransference*. Northvale, NJ: Jason Aronson.

Krystal, H. (1988). *Integration and healing*. Hillsdale, NJ: Analytic Press.

Krystal, H. (1988). *Massive psychic trauma*. New York: International Universtiy Ben.

Levenson, R. W. & Ruef, A. M. (1997). Psychological aspects of emotional knowledge. In W. Ickes (Ed.), *Emapathic accuracy* (pp. 44–73). New York: Guilford Publications.

Pearlman, L. & Saakvitne, K. (1995). *Trauma and the therapist*. New York: Norton.

Racker, H. (1968). *Transference and countertransference*. New York: International Universities Press.

Schore, A. N. (2003a). *Affect dysregulation and disorders of the self*. New York: Norton.

Schore, A. N. (2003b). *Affect regulation and the repair of the self*. New York: Norton.

Tansey, M. J. & Burke, W. F. (1989). *Understanding countertransference*. Hillsdale, NJ: Erlbaum.

van der Kolk, B., McFarlane, A. C. & Weisaeth, L. (1997). *Traumatic stress*. New York: Guilford Publications.

Wilson, J. P. (2002, October). *The abyss experience and the trauma complex: A Jungian perspective of post-traumatic stress disorder and dissociation*. Presentation at St. Joseph's University, Terrorism and Weapons of Mass Destruction, Philadelphia, PA.

Wilson, J. P., Friedman, M. J. & Lindy, J. D. (2001). *Treating psychological trauma and PTSD*. New York: Guilford Publications.

Wilson, J. P. & Lindy, J. (1994). *Countertransference in the treatment of PTSD*. New York: Guilford Publications.

7

Anxiety and Defensiveness in the Trauma Therapist

The literature on transference and countertransference in psychoanalysis has long established the importance of understanding how the analyst is affected during the course of treatment (Wolstein, 1988). In a similar way, research and clinical studies of PTSD, and intensive work with trauma patients, have described the various ways that therapists, first responders, counselors, crisis debriefers, nurses, physicians and others are impacted by the nature of trauma work. In fact, it is not so much a question of whether or not trauma therapists are emotionally affected in their professional role, but rather in what ways they are affected and for how long. Given the immersion into the world of traumatized individuals, how will the affects stirred by such powerful exposure influence the nature of the therapist's capacity to remain empathically attuned, professionally competent and optimally functional?

Since empathy is the "psychobiological capacity to experience another person's state of being and phenomenological perspective at any given moment in time" (Wilson & Lindy, 1994, p. 27), it is inevitable that empathic processes will cause the therapist, through empathic identification, to experience the inner turmoil and psychic states of clients. It is precisely for this reason that we have conceptualized the nature of the balance beam between modalities of empathic attunement and empathic strains. How do therapists maintain their own sense of balance and equilibrium during the course of post-traumatic therapy? How does the experience of anxiety and defensiveness impinge on empathic balance?

Empathic attunement, openness to the experiences of others, and understanding the nature of patients' internal working models of personal trauma demand the ability to "get inside" their world and view the inner set of traumatic memories and the dysregulated affects that accompany them. By empathic immersion into the psychic inner core of ego-spaces, the therapist develops an acute sense of what the original trauma was like for the patient and how it changed the latter's life. In an analogous way, this immersion is like watching a movie on a wide screen accompanied by realistic stereophonic "surround sound" and palpable sensory perceptions of smell, touch, taste, movement and emotions. Exposure to the intricacies of the patient's trauma stories, such as those in the case histories of Teresa, the Bosnian widow whose husband was tortured to death, and the young Marines Corps combat veteran of Vietnam, inevitably result in affect dysregulation in the therapist, not unlike the affect dysregulations experienced by the patient during and after the trauma, but to a lesser degree of severity.

Affect dysregulation in the therapist is a precursor of states of anxiety and defensiveness (Schore, 2003b). States of affect dysregulation are dynamically associated with empathic identification. The power of trauma transference is such that it causes states of emotional disequilibrium, a change from stasis, and is a signal affect (Tansey & Burke, 1989) of dysregulation which sets in motion a series of psychological effects, including challenges to personal world views, beliefs, ideologies and systems of value. A similar observation has been made by Pearlman and Saakvitne (1995) who state,

> Strong affects challenge a therapist's identity, both personal and professional. A therapist with an identity as tough and resilient may feel distressed and ashamed to find himself undone with grief or identificatory feelings, likely to arise in clients who are victims of harsh punishment. A trauma therapist whose work is based on his capacity for hope in the face of his client's despair may be shaken when he finds himself joining with the client's hopelessness in an unconscious transference reaction. (p. 318)

When considered in a larger perspective of emotional responsiveness, empathy and defenses, it becomes clear that affect dysregulation requires identification, modulation, control and management of information during post-traumatic therapy (see Figure 7.5). The question arises, then, as to the clues to different types of experienced affect dysregulation, and the psychological processes used by the therapist to contain and use them constructively. Stated differently, what are the signs and symptoms of anxiety and defensiveness in the therapist? Are there special risk factors for therapists who choose to work with trauma and PTSD? Do signs and symptoms of anxiety and defensiveness have diagnostic and clinical therapeutic significance, in terms of Type I and Type II CTR and the modalities of empathic attunement and empathic strains?

The foregoing questions are not necessarily new ones; they have their roots of origin in early psychodynamic perspectives on affects, transference and countertransference. For example, Mabel Blake Cohen (1952) stated,

> ...recent studies on countertransference have included in their concepts attitudes of the therapist that are both conscious and unconscious; attitudes that are *responses* both to real and to fantasized attributes of the patient;

attitudes that are *stimulated by unconscious needs of the analyst* and attitudes that are stimulated by *sudden outbursts of affect on the part of the patient*...The common factor in the above responses is the *presence of anxiety in the therapist*—whether recognized in awareness or defended against and kept out of awareness. (p. 69, italics ours)

A similar position has been presented by Karen J. Maroda (1991) in her book, *The Power of Countertransference*:

A therapist *feels anxiety* when a patient needs a particular response and, in provoking the desired response, he *accidentally threatens* the therapist, *overwhelming his defenses* [cf. empathic strain}...ideally the therapist only experiences anxiety transiently in a session and is able to recover his *equilibrium* through insight, thereby giving a perspective on the true situation. (p. 148, italics ours)

Maroda (1991) is suggesting that anxiety is experienced when the patient "accidentally" threatens the therapist and disrupts the latter's equilibrium, thereby creating empathic strain. However, with insight into the "transient" state of disequilibrium, the therapist will regain composure and, presumably, empathic attunement. Maroda (1991) seems to be echoing the earlier position of Heinrich Racker (1957), in his classic and widely cited paper, "The Meanings and Uses of Countertransference," published in the *Psychoanalytic Quarterly* (26, pp. 303–357).

As noted earlier, Racker coined the phrase "dual unfolding process" between the therapist and the patient, each manifesting affects, defenses and "themes" associated with the specific course of treatment with its nuances, character and individual style:

Every transference situation provokes a countertransference situation, which arises out of the analyst's identification of himself with the analysand's (internal) objects...*these countertransference situations cannot be avoided*; certainly they should not be avoided *if full understanding is to be achieved*... (p. 167, cited in Wolstein, 1988, italics ours)

What does a "full understanding" mean? To achieve it, as indicated by Racker, implies that the therapist is able to modulate CTR reactions which are "provoked" by the patient's transference. Racker seems to be implying that the CTR reaction contains useful information for the analyst, and that being "provoked," in and of itself, is meaningful to understanding the interpersonal dynamics occurring during treatment. Alternatively, we can think of this process as suggesting that one analyst's "provocation" by a patient may be another's "pacification," since there are distinct personality differences in therapists which influence the way in which transference is received and processed (Hedges, 1992; Wolstein, 1988).

Individual differences in responses to traumatic transferences have figured prominently in Pearlman and Saatvikne's (1995) analysis of vicarious traumatization in post-traumatic therapy. The constructivist self-development theory (McCann & Pearlman, 1990; Pearlman & Saatvikne, 1995) proposes five classes of variables which serve as mediators of trauma processing by the therapist: (1) ideological frame of reference; (2) self-capacities; (3) ego-resources; (4) psychological needs for safety, trust, esteem, intimacy and control; and (5) memory system capacities. The authors suggest that these factors filter vicarious trauma exposures during treatment and, in turn, are affected by them. These five factors are also areas where psychological defenses will operate to protect the therapist when vicarious traumatization poses challenges to cherished beliefs, to the self-image of the therapist as a competent person, or to overwhelmed ego-resources. In describing psychological defenses in the treatment of trauma and PTSD, Pearlman and Saatvikne (1995) state,

> The therapist will experience his powerful emotional responses in the context of his own self-capacities. A therapist who is uncomfortable with strong feelings in general or certain feelings in particular, or whose *affect tolerance is exceeded* by specific feelings will draw upon his familiar *protective defenses.* These defenses can *compromise* his ability to remain *affectievly* available and genuine to himself or his client. (p. 319, italics ours)

This passage is consistent with our analysis of the importance of understanding how affect dysregulation, generated by TST by the patient, sets up the processes of empathic strain as clinical skills in sustaining empathic attunement are challenged. The intrapsychic tension, generated by the balance beam of the opposing forces of empathic attunement and empathic strain, leads to anxiety and defensiveness if the balance beam tilts suddenly or gradually to the side of empathic strain, leaving empathic attunement "up-ended," "in the air," like a child on a teeter-totter with its much heavier parent touching the ground at the opposite end. Pearlman and Saatvikne (1995) have reached a similar conclusion from the constructivist self-development theory:

> *Many trauma therapists move defensively* into a stance of *emotional vulnerability which requires affective numbing.* The denial of any affects that contradict a defensive identity then prevents other protective or supportive measures. One cannot soothe or protect oneself from *affects* one *denies* having.... A therapist may feel horrified when he feels little sadness or compassion in response to a client's traumatic memories, experiences, or self-destructive behaviors. Another therapist may be appalled at his feelings of rage, arousal or sadism in response to a trauma client. (p. 320, italics ours)

How do trauma therapists "move defensively" into states of affective numbing or emotional anesthesia? What is it, precisely, that so overwhelms their ego-resources and adaptive coping patterns that they "switch-off" feelings in order to deal with their patients and their powerful trauma stories? Why should trauma work, PTSD and the affective intensity of TSTT cause a cessation of empathic attunement? What is the defensive and/or adaptive function of psychic numbing?

PSYCHIC NUMBING AS DEFENSIVE ARMOR

It is instructive to note that the term *psychic numbing* was developed by Robert J. Lifton (1967) in his pioneering work with survivors of the first atomic bombing at Hiroshima, Japan. Lifton observed that, in response to the pervasiveness of death, destruction and historically unprecedented massive catastrophe, most Japanese survivors (cf. *Hibaksha*) experienced psychic numbing. As characterized by Lifton, psychic numbing was an automatic and adaptive response for the survivors of the atomic bomb, who were immediately immersed into an abyss of Hell: death, thousands of radiation burned and mutilated bodies, dying persons crying for help, and the total destruction of the environs of the large island-bound city. The world and culture of Hiroshima, as the survivors had known it, no longer existed. To survive in the immediate aftermath required a numbed, automatic state of functioning, in order to face the uncertain future and the perils of radiation exposure and sickness whose effects were little understood at the time but caused suffering and death on a daily basis for decades (Lifton, 1967).

In later clarifications and elaborations on the functions of psychic numbing, Lifton delineated its various forms in his book, *The Life of the Self* (1976). Here he identified that there are degrees of psychic numbing, as there are degrees of anger, joy, sadness and depression:

> Psychic numbing is a form of desensitization; it refers to an incapacity to feel or to confront certain kinds of experience due to the blocking or absence of inner forms or imagery that can connect with such experiences (Lifton, 1976, p. 27)

Thus, psychic numbing is not an "all or none" phenomenon which switches "on" and "off" like a light. Extending Lifton's definition, we find psychic numbing to be multidimensional and pertaining to (1) emotions; (2) psychoformative cognitive processes; (3) capacity for self-monitoring; (4) capacity to experience affects; (5) cessation in empathic attunement; and (6) loss of capacity for genuine interpersonal relations. When these dimensions of psychic numbing are considered in the context of post-traumatic therapy, it is apparent that the "movement" into psychic numbing described by Pearlman and Saakvitne is a defensive posture to attempt to control and modulate affective dysregulations associated with feelings of vulnerability, anxiety and uncertainty in the process of treating trauma patients. Moreover, the presence of psychic numbing in the therapist will inevitably lead to a rupture in empathy and Type I or Type II CTR (Wilson & Lindy, 1994). Psychically numb therapists will be ineffective in staying attuned to their patients; they will "miss" subtle cues and interpersonal patterns of behavior that are being "projected" in the transference. In some instances, the presence of *psychic numbing in the therapist* may be a "mirror reflection" of *psychically numbed patients*, wherein the therapist unwittingly and unconsciously takes on the same "defensive armor" as his patients—somewhat akin to a knight of the Middle Ages donning his metal armor body suit and protective chain mail mesh to go into battle, carefully reserving the protective helmet to the last moment for final adornment.

Psychic numbing, like ancient full metal body armor, limits flexibility, mobility and capacity to see and hear effectively that which confronts the therapist. Its functional value is protection against attack and vulnerability to injury, and is of limited usefulness. Prolonged use of psychic numbing results in states of fatigue, exhaustion, somatic complaints, ineffectiveness at work, dysphoria, malaise, loss of sensuality and interpersonal sensitivity (Lifton, 1976; Wilson, Friedman, & Lindy, 2001). Psychic numbing impedes accurate information decoding of trauma transferences from the patient. Psychic numbing is not only a defensive response to feeling overwhelmed by taxing stressors of an emotional nature, but it is also associated with distinct negative styles of personality in therapists.

WOLSTEIN'S TYPOLOGY OF ANALYSTS' PERSONALITY TRAITS, DEFENSIVENESS AND INTERPERSONAL STYLES

How are personality traits related to anxiety and defensiveness in therapists? In an attempt to understand the complex dynamics of countertransference, Benjamin Wolstein (1988) states,

> Since no two analysts are identical, we are compelled to seek out and make intelligible the differences among them, their *modes of experience, value orientations* and *styles of therapeutic activity*…. The observations are based on *dominant personality traits,* and it is quite possible that a specific analyst may fall into more than one category … these traits are descriptive not only of analysts at work but also in their every day living. (pp. 225–226, italics ours)

Wolstein's departure point is to identify a limited number of "dominant personality traits" that characterize the domain of analytic practitioners. He classifies five personality typologies which are germane to our understanding of anxiety and defenses in post-traumatic therapies. These five typologies are labeled by Wolstein as: (I) overprotective nurturing; (II) aggressive dependency; (III) model adjustment (narcissistic); (IV) obsessive criticism; and (V) detachment. We will briefly summarize each of these personality typologies, and then relate them to modalities of empathic attunement, empathic strain and Type I and Type II CTR.

Type I—Overprotective Nurturing

Wolstein's first personality typology is described as an overprotective nurturing analyst, who, Wolstein believes, has an usual ability "to establish nurturing contact" with his or her patients. However, the psychological origin of such therapists' nurturing capacity and sensitivity to patients derives, in part, from their own need to be cared for, protected, secured, and involved in trusting, predictable relationships. Unconsciously, such therapists seek out dependency fulfilling relationships. In their professional role they "give to get," displaying the oral-dependent counterphobic reaction to fixated infantile oral conflicts (Erikson, 1968). As part of this personality style, the overprotective dependent therapist nurtures his or her patients by creating a "shield-like cocoon" of security which eventually leads to problems in the course of analysis. The overprotective nurturing personality style is best characterized by strong traits of dependency which mold the tapestry of the analytic situation. In our view, such therapists are prone to Type II CTR, overidentification, and will experience empathic strain because of enmeshment tendencies. Their mode of empathic attunement corresponds to empathic inconsistency, in which there is overidealization, undermodulated affect and persistent styles of disequilibrium which reflect these therapists' personality dynamics.

Type II—Aggressive Dependency

Wolstein's second personality typology is characterized by "aggressive dependency or exploitativeness" (p. 229). These analysts present a façade of an aggressive, no nonsense, "get down to business" attitude. Wolstein uses the description "aggressive dependency" because such therapists have strong dependency needs, and may act assertively and exploitatively with patients to assume control of therapeutic processes in the service of their needs. Due to deep-seated, unfulfilled dependency needs, these therapists experience anxiety, threat and distress when their efforts to direct treatment do not succeed. The aggressive dependent personality style is associated with ego-defenses of denial, resulting in the therapist failing to see that his or her needs for intimacy and warmth are being frustrated during the treatment process.

According to Wolstein, once the therapist's defenses are activated by the patient's demands for intimacy, the analyst either detaches and withdraws or runs the risk of acting in manipulative, exploitative ways. It is for this reason that reliable therapeutic detachment is *incongruent* with this personality style, and sets up intrapsychic conflict. Thus, there develops alternating motifs of detachment, and aggressively initiated dependency relations characterize the countertransference. This personality style corresponds to a Type I (avoidance) modality of CTR with empathic strains being associated with a predisposition to detachment, withdrawal and repression of personal needs. Such a therapeutic method is strongly associated with the empathic attunement modality of "empathic insufficiency," characterized by pseudo-empathy, exploitativeness, distancing and inadequacy.

Type III—Modeled Adjustment (Narcissistic)

Wolstein's third personality typology is described as "model adjustment" which is a misnomer, since Wolstein clarifies that he is referring to a narcissistic personality orientation. The term *model adjustment* was used to characterize the therapist who appears to be a model analyst when, in fact, he or she suffers from insufficiencies in self-esteem, and exhibits many of the attributes of narcissistic personality disorder, such as seeking adulation and recognition from others (i.e., mirror hungry personality, Wolfe, 1990), an inflated sense of self-worth and grandiosity, especially in his or her ability to dazzle patients (and self) with interpretive scenarios based on minimal data. Wolstein notes: "This is the man of small personal feeling who finds signs of his intuitive gift in his ability to work out and apply intricate interpretive schemes to minimal clues" (p. 279). The narcissistic "model" analyst is driven by his or her personality dynamics to succeed, which limits his or her depth of genuine empathic attunement, or as Wolstein states: "he has *very little feeling* ... for personality as an integrated organic unity moving towards him and trying to experience him" (p. 235).

The self-inflated grandiose self-image of the narcissistic personality typology not only reflects simulation of the outward appearance of being a "model analyst," but also hides deep insecurity, personal doubts, and feelings of inadequacy and inferiority. In fact, he unthinkingly or sometimes brazenly "requires the patient to submit unconscious material to substantiate his flawed theoretical conceptions" (p. 236). The self-contentedness of the narcissistic analyst renders him indifferent to the patient's acceptance of his interpretation since he, by virtue of being a professional analyst, is above reproach, rejection or retribution. As a consequence, his narcissistic defenses against inadequacy, low self-esteem and self-doubt are associated with little insight into his own CTR processes. This personality-based therapeutic style is associated with Type I CTR, avoidance and empathic strains of withdrawal. This therapist's primary mode of empathic attunement is empathic insufficiency.

Type IV—Obsessive Criticism

The fourth personality style is distinguished by obsessive identity traits and rigid, overcontrolled forms of cognitive style and information processing. The besettingly critical analyst is detail-oriented and perfectionistic. He is rigid in analytic technique and compulsively insistent on adherence to protocol in a structured, orderly and conformist fashion. The obsessive analyst is precisionistic, and demands that he carefully scrutinize himself, being scrupulous to avoid engaging in any unseemingly unconventional actions in his role as analyst. This therapist firmly and rigorously compartmentalizes his own needs and conflicts, viewing them as unrelated to treatment. He is prone to isolate affect, and to intellectualize and focus on technical performance rather than empathic flow with the patient.

The overreliance on technique, methodology and the maintenance of role propriety, in a rigidly governed manner, tends to make the obsessive analyst insensitive and without genuine empathic attunement to the patients. Such analysts are afraid of strong emotional outbursts from their patients, and are easily disarmed and threatened by unexpected displays of emotion, particularly anger and intense transference reactions. The obsessive personality typology is generally uncomfortable with feelings, and is prone to countertransference distortions. Their ego-defenses are part of a cyclical style of coping with threats or demands made by their patients. As the therapist's rigidity (and detachment) increases, the patient makes demands in a more assertive and insistent manner, while the analyst further detaches, analyzes, overintellectualizes and rigidly adheres to technique, being out of touch with his or her own psychological processes. This personality typology is associated with Type I CTR and types of empathic strain characterized by withdrawal and repression. The predominant modality of empathic attunement is empathic weakness with strong defensive controls, numbing, withdrawal and repression.

Type V—Detachment

The fifth personality style is note for detachment in the analytic process. The detached analyst has excellent powers of observation and adherence to technique. Such analysts firmly believe in and rely upon the "blank façade" in treatment. Their aloof, uncommitted approach to clinical treatment precludes an active collaboration with patients and eventually creates conflicts, except for the most compliant of patients. These dispassionate analysts are nondisclosing and reveal little of themselves to their patients who, in turn, search for clues as to how to approach and engage the analyst in more intimate ways. This therapeutic stance of aloofness and self-containment lead some patients to act out, to test the limits of the tightly guarded style of clinical interaction. As part of their defensively guarded mode of patient interaction, these uninvolved analysts misconstrue their aloofness with objectivity; this leads to confrontation with non-compliant and more assertive patients who want to connect with the "person behind the mask."

The detached analyst does not have the characterological strength to have an open, egalitarian relationship with patients. Such analysts believe, instead, that it is the patient's therapeutic task to create a positive emotional climate and that they (the therapists), by rigidly maintaining a "blank screen" facade and cool detachment, will compel the patient to manifest more transference material for interpretation, thus reinforcing and justifying the detached clinical style. This personality typology is associated with Type I CTR and withdrawal modes of empathic strain. The analyst's predominant modality of empathic attunement is distancing, characterized by counterphobic behaviors, detachment and emotional isolation.

In the way of a summary overview, Wolstein (1988) believes that the personality styles of analysts are the product of their own developmental experiences, conflicts and ego-defensive styles. Consistent with Racker's (1957) position, the patient's transference can provoke defenses in the analyst, setting in motion an array of defensive tactics, strategies and counterdefensive maneuvers. It is the presence of anxiety that provides the clue to CTRs:

> The easiest way for an analyst to identify countertransference distortions is his observation of the *usual signs of anxiety in himself*. They may run the wide gamut from *transient anxiety reactions, the continuation of an emotion from one session to another and its recurrence at the end of the day*, to the point *where his anxiety reactions require serious attention, to acting out and identifying the patient as reminiscent of a particularly difficult or disturbing person in his own personal history*. (p. 254, italics ours)

Wolstein's (1988) typology of personality styles and their association with countertransference modalities is useful in several ways. First, it identifies personality-based patterns of therapists which strongly influence the nature, quality and adequacy of the therapeutic dyad. Second, it provides sufficient description of the therapeutic process to discern modalities of empathic attunement, empathic strain and countertransference. Third, it permits a meta-theoretical conceptual analysis of the underlying structural and process dimensions presented in chapter 4. For example, with sufficient data on the analyst's style of interaction over a sufficient period of time, these personality-based differences in behavior could be compared to the 10 dimensions of process discussed in chapter 4: (1) the therapist's affective reactions; (2) boundary management dynamics; (3) countertransference regulation and management; (4) therapeutic alliance maintenance; (5) pattern of empathic attunement vs. empathic strain; (6) clinical skill level; (7) assessment of treatment progress; (8) cognition and formulation of patient's symptoms; (9) formulation of treatment places and target objectives; and (10) determination of treatment efficacy and outcomes.

In the way of a summary analysis, Figure 7.1 illustrates the relationship between Wolstein's typology of personality traits and their association with empathic attunements, empathic strains and countertransference. It is evident from this figure that 80% of countertransference styles are Type I patterns of avoidance. Only the overprotective nurturer warrants a Type II (overidentification) classification of enmeshment and reciprocal dependency. In terms of empathic attunement, the most prevalent modality manifest is empathic insufficiency which takes the form of pseudo-empathy (narcissistic type), distancing (detachment type), and insensitivity/desensitization (aggressive dependency type). The only Type II countertransference is evident in the form of empathic inconsistency which involves enmeshment, reciprocal dependency, states of disequilibrium, compensatory and counterphobic behaviors in the personality style of the overprotective nurturer.

These findings match Ernest Wolfe's (1990) observations, namely, that an analyst's personal need for excessive mirroring may result from: (1) the patient's *overidealization* of the therapist; (2) the therapist's inability to meaningfully connect with the patient due to empathic insufficiencies; or (3) the dysregulated affects experienced by the therapist. In post-traumatic

Personality Trait Typology	Modes of Empathic Attunement	Modes of Empathic Strain	Type I or Type II Countertransference
I. Overprotective Nurturer	Empathic Inconsistency	Empathic Enmeshment	Type II
II. Aggressive Dependency	Empathic Insufficiency	Empathic Withdrawal	Type I
III. Narcissistic (Model Adjustment)	Empathic Insufficiency	Empathic Withdrawal	Type I
IV. Obsessive-Critic	Empathic Weakness	Empathic Withdrawal/ Repression	Type I
V. Detached	Empathic Insufficiency	Empathic Withdrawal	Type I

Figure 7.1 Wolstein's (1988) typology of therapists personality traits and their relation to empathic attunement, empathic strain and countertransference. Copyright John P. Wilson, 2003.

therapy, the intensity and nature of the trauma survivor can readily stimulate the need for "excessive mirroring" since the survivor's experiences are those of enduring the horrors of interpersonal abuse, war, disasters and the events that make them fragile, vulnerable, resilient or heroic patients who have encountered the dark forces of the abyss and survived (Wilson, 2003).

ANXIETY AND DEFENSIVENESS IN THE THERAPIST DURING TREATMENT OF THE PATIENT

The therapeutic dyad is a microcosm of human interpersonal relationships. Beyond the constraints imposed by professional role boundaries, what transpires in psychotherapy recapitulates social transactions in naturalistic settings. The constraints imposed by professional role boundaries, and the reliance on more or less structured techniques of inquiry, govern treatment approaches which, in turn, create a unique environment in which the observing study and analysis of psychological problems occurs.

Psychodynamic approaches to treating emotional problems, in which anxiety is a central feature, focus on the world of inner experiences (Wolfe, 1990). Behaviorally oriented treatment approaches center more exclusively on external manifestations of emotional problems than on inner experiences. We believe that the two foci are not mutually exclusive, especially in the understanding and treatment of trauma and PTSD. For example, how can one understand the trauma of incest, rape or terrorist bombing attacks without access to the patient's inner world where nightmares, traumatic memories, dysregulated affects, thoughts of suicide and an abandonment of religious faith result after victimization?

Moreover, if one were to rely *only* on overt external manifestations of PTSD symptoms in victims of trauma, they would not look radically different in most respects from persons without the disorder, except for those episodic occasions when symptoms are overt such as dissociative behaviors, flashbacks, trauma specific startle reactions, disturbing trauma related nightmares, or unusual phobic behaviors related to the trauma experience, as seen in agoraphobia associated with disasters, groups of people (e.g., combat platoon) and open public spaces (e.g., a terrorist suicide attack). To state this question differently, if one were to randomly sample PTSD patients with different trauma histories, and videotape their behavior in normal social interaction in a laboratory setting, could they be distinguished from a matched set of cohorts without a history of PTSD? For example, could undergraduate university students tell the difference between PTSD patients and non-PTSD patients by watching a videotape social interaction or by actually observing an "in vivo" interaction?

ANTIPODAL EMPATHY: A LOOK AT THE THERAPIST'S INNER WORLD

We are in agreement with Kohut (1977) that empathy is a clinical and scientific tool that permits entry into the inner sanctum of the psyche in all of its structural complexity. As Ernest Wolfe (1990) noted: "data obtained by vicarious introspection (= empathy) can be combined with introspective data to get a more complex picture of the psychological world in depth" (p. 33). Wolfe suggests that empathy has three primary purposes: (1) to define an approach to observation and treatment; (2) to obtain data by using empathy as a "microscope" with different levels of magnifying power; and (3) to provide a communication style of interaction which is sustaining to patients and reassures them that their inner world and problems are understood. To quote Wolfe (1990),

> Since the self, in order to stay structurally intact, must be embedded in a matrix of sustaining relationships with self-objects—that is, self-object experiences—the *vicissitudes of self-object relations become the focus* of interest both for the study of the etiology of disorders of the self and for the therapeutic interventions to ameliorate these disorders. (p. 38, italics ours)

This passage is particularly relevant to our understanding of the relationship of empathic attunement, empathic strain and defensiveness in the therapist during treatment of trauma and PTSD patients. By analyzing the "other side of the desk," that is, the therapist or care provider, we can use empathy to discern the nature of the therapist's inner world. Traditionally, this phenomenon has been discussed under the technical rubric as transference—countertransference. However, it is more than that, since it entails using the same power of empathic magnification, or clinical-scientific skills, to enter the inner sanctum of the therapist's world and thereby capture the full range of his internal working models of the process of therapy *and* himself as a self-process. In this respect, we need to study the vicissitudes and metamorphic changes in the structure of the analyst's psyche *in vivo* during treatment and afterwards as cognitive-affective processing occurs. This idea of applying analytic scrutiny to therapists was proposed a half century ago by M.B. Cohen (1952), who stated,

> The study of countertransference responses provides a rich field for the further investigation of the doctor-patient relationship in psychoanalysis and intensive psychotherapy. *This is made more feasible by the possibility of using recordings and interviews both as research tools and as training adjuncts.* As the therapist increases his *awareness* of the nature of his participation with the patient—both on the basis of his own *personal needs and on the basis of the roles cast for him by the patient*—his therapeutic management of the interaction can become more precise and the range of neurotic problems that he is able to tackle can be expected to increase. (p. 82, italics ours)

PSYCHOBIOLOGICAL PROFILE OF HIGH VS. LOW EMPATHY IN THE THERAPIST

When reflecting on this passage by M. B. Cohen (1952), it is helpful to remember that her insights were made before the advent of videotape technology and before other more advanced technical equipment was available. Given current technological research tools, virtually all aspects of a therapist's activity could be examined in detail—utilizing MRIs, PET scans, physiological monitors, pupil scans, postural changes, muscle tension, cardiovascular functions, real-time verbal recordings and psychometric assessments. The "feasibility" suggested by Cohen is now a reality of scientific opportunity to use multiple methods of research in studying the therapist's empathic capacities.

Is there, in fact, a scientifically discernible state of "high empathy" as described in chapter 5? If empathy is the means of introspection to knowledge of inner psychological states, what are the quantitative and qualitative dimensions of empathy? For example, we have stated that high empathy is characterized by such attributes as precise signal decoding, accurate tracking of clients' internal states, meticulous signal detection, phasic synchrony in physiological states, focal receptivity, verbal response cadence and timing, etc. Clearly, these are operationally measurable constructs which could be assessed in a variety of clinical and experimental settings to gain portals of entrance into the therapist's psychological space. The data for such research efforts will eventually enable identification of the psychobiological basis of empathy, and to understand its role more precisely in the treatment of psychological disorders, especially PTSD as a prolonged stress response pattern. In this sense, it should be possible to measure and construct psychological profiles of empathic ability as a psychobiological propensity in personality.

SIGNS AND SYMPTOMS OF TRAUMA ANXIETY AND DEFENSIVENESS IN THE THERAPIST

In this section clinical data relevant to understanding the signs and symptoms of anxiety and defense in the trauma therapist is reviewed. In a more focused way, this data is used to highlight the process of affect dysregulation in the therapist during the course of post-traumatic therapy. The review bears in mind Allan Schore's (2003a) conclusion that

> an understanding that the *therapist's affect tolerance is a critical factor determining the range, types, and intensities of emotions that are explored or disavowed in the transference—countertransference relationship in the therapeutic alliance.* (p. 281, italics ours)

Figures 7.2, 7.3 and 7.4 offer a summary of the signs and symptoms of anxiety and defensiveness in the therapist, and show their correspondence to modes of empathic attunement, empathic strains and countertransference processes. Finally, Figure 7.5 illustrates the dynamic relationship of affect dysregulation, anxiety states, coping and defense in post-traumatic therapies.

The experience of anxiety and defensiveness during post-traumatic therapy is expectable and universal, especially given the context of the treatment focus. The idea that the analyst's level of anxiety and defensiveness is a potential problem in countertransference is not new, and has been the subject of extensive investigation. For example, in 1952, M. B. Cohen wrote a remarkable and insightful paper entitled "Counter-

Signs of Anxiety and Defensiveness in Analyst (1952)	Modes of Empathic Strain (A) and Type I or Type II (B)** Countertransference Reactions		
	Mode A	CTR B	
1. Unreasonable dislike for patient	III	I	(disdain, repression)
2. Failure to identify with patient	III	I	(detachment, withdrawal)
3. Nonresponsiveness to emotional distress of patient	II	I	(distance, avoidance)
4. Overwhelmed by patient's problems	I	II	(disequilibrium)
5. Excessive liking of patient	III	II	(enmeshment)
6. Dreads therapy session/uncomfortable during session	II	I	(fear, anxiety)
7. Preoccupation with patient outside office	III	II	(overinvolvement)
8. Inattention, problems of concentration, drowsiness, sleepy	II	I	(avoidance, denial, withdrawal)
9. Preoccupation with own (personal) affairs	II	I	(avoidance, withdrawal)
10. Analyst has problems with time management (late to session)	II	I	(avoidance, withdrawal)
11. Argumentative with patient	III	II	(overinvolvement, defensive)
12. Defensive with patient; feels vulnerable	III	II	(overidentification, defensive)
13. Countertransference distortion	II	I	(withdrawal, misperception of dynamics)
14. Analyst elicits affect; prods patient	III	II	(enmeshment)
15. Overconcerned with confidentiality	III	II	(enmeshment)
16. Oversympathetic due to mistreatment by authority of patient	III	II	(overidentification)
17. Urge to help in acting	I	II	(overidentification, prosocial, disequilibrium)
18. Patient appears in analyst's dreams	III	II	(overidentification)

*Mabel Blake Cohen (1952). "Counter-transference and anxiety." Psychiatry, 15, pp. 231–243.
** After Wilson and Lindy (1994).

Figure 7.2 Mabel Blake Cohen (1952) anxiety and defensiveness in analyst during treatment of patient. Copyright John P. Wilson, 2002.

Signs, Symptoms and Behaviors	Modes of Empathic Strain and Type I or Type II Countertransference Reactions		
	Mode (A)	CTR (B)	
1. Agreeing with the patient	III	III	(overidentification, enmeshment)
2. Detachment (any form)	III	I	(withdrawal, avoidance)
3. Withdrawing from patient	I, II	I	(withdrawal, repression)
4. Overly critical	I	I	(avoidance, distancing)
5. Overly silent	II	I	(avoidance, withdrawal)
6. Overtly/covertly judgmental	I	I	(avoidance, distancing)
7. Overtly/covertly judgmental	I	I	(avoidance, distancing)
8. Passive aggression in repeating interpretation	I	I	(avoidance, repression, anger)
9. Overintellectualization to intense affect	I	I	(avoidance, withdrawal)
10. Cancel appointments	I	I	(avoidance, distancing, withdrawal)
11. Forget appointments	I	I	(avoidance, distancing, withdrawal)
12. Reschedule, double schedule appointments	I	I	(avoidance, distancing, withdrawal)
13. Persistent anger	III	II	(overidentification, enmeshment)
14. Persistent idealization	III	II	(overidentification, enmeshment)
15. Failure to confront nonpayment of fees	II	I	(avoidance, repression)
16. Feeling "hooked" or "sucked on"	III	II	(enmeshment, loss of boundary)
17. Fear of being out of control	IV	II	(disequilibrium, unmodulated affect)
18. Atypical nervousness	IV	II	(disequilibrium, vulnerability)
19. Nightmares about patient	III	II	(enmeshment, over-identification)
20. Erotic/love feelings towards patient	III	II	(enmeshment, over-involvement)
21. Refusal to answer reasonable questions	I	I	(avoidance, withdrawal)

See chapter 4 for Types of Empathic Strains (I–IV)

Figure 7.3 Signs, symptoms and behaviors associated with anxiety and defensiveness in psychodynamic therapy, Karen J. Maroda (1991). Copyright John P. Wilson, 2003.

transference and Anxiety" in which she proposed five therapeutic situations likely to produce anxiety and countertransference:

> The main situations in the doctor-patient relationship that undermine the therapeutic role and therapy, and may result in anxiety in the therapist, can be listed as follows: (1) when the doctor is *helpless* to affect the patients' memories; (2) when the doctor is treated continually as an *object of fear, hatred or contempt*; (3) when the patient calls on the doctor for advice or reassurance as evidence of his professional competence or interest in the patient; (4) when the patient attempts to establish a relationship of *romantic love* with the doctor; and (5) when the patient calls on the doctor for other intimacy. (1952, 1988, p. 73, italics ours)

I. **PHYSIOLOGICAL AND PHYSICAL REACTIONS**
 Symptoms of increased ANS arousal (e.g., heart palpitations, muscle tension)
 Somatic reactions to trauma story or therapy as a contextual process (e.g., stomach pain)
 Sleep disturbances; nightmares of patient's trauma
 Agitation, inability to relax, on edge, hypersensitivity
 Inattention, drowsiness, avoidance reactions, yawning, rubbing eyes, sleepiness
 Uncontrolled and unintended displays of emotion (e.g., tears, heavy breathing, sighing)
 Isochronicity: physiological parallelism to affective state, client (anger, sadness, tension)

II. **EMOTIONAL REACTIONS**
 Irritability, annoyance, disdain, or resentment towards client
 Anxiety and fear
 Depression, helpless, sense of hopelessness, futility
 Anger, rage, hostility, passive aggression
 Detachment, denial, avoidance, numbing, desires for aloneness and isolation
 Sadistic/masochistic feelings
 Voyeuristic and sexualized feelings
 Horror, disgust, dread, loathing, terror
 Confusion, psychic overload, overwhelmed, foggy after session
 Guilt, shame, embarrassment
 Sadness, grief, sorrow
 Fatigue, exhaustion, feeling "drained," "spent," "wasted," "depleted"

III. **PSYCHOLOGICAL REACTIONS**
 Detachment reactions based on defenses of intellectualization, rationalization, isolation, denial, minimization, fantasy
 Overidentification based on defenses of projection, introjection, denial, altruism

IV. **SIGNS AND BEHAVIORAL SYMPTOMS OF CTRs THAT MAY BE CONSCIOUS OR UNCONSCIOUS**
 Preoccupation with patient's trauma history, dreams, presentation during treatment
 Rescue fantasies: problem "fixer," hero, rescuer, "dragon slayer," "white knight," good parent, etc.
 Forgetting, lapse of attention, parapraxes
 Leave therapeutic role stance of empathy (i.e., loss of empathic attunement)
 Overhostility, anger toward client, criticalness
 Relief when client misses appointment or wish that client not attend session
 Repeated scheduling problems by therapist
 Denial of feelings and/or need for supervision/consultation
 Narcissistic belief in role of being specialist in PTSD (i.e., superior skills, grandiose fantasies, gifted healer, etc.)
 Excessive concern/identification with client (e.g., take trauma impact "home")
 Psychic numbing or emotional constriction; de-sexualization, loss of sensuality and interpersonal sensitivity
 Self-medication as numbing (i.e., use of alcohol, etc. to reduce affect and preoccupation)
 Loss of boundaries during therapy
 Preoccupation with referring client or terminating treatment

Figure 7.4 Factors indicative of CTRs in therapist/helper. Copyright John P. Wilson and Jacob D. Lindy, 1994; John P. Wilson, 2003.

This passage is germane to our focus on empathy and countertransference, because it highlights the situations likely to produce anxiety: namely, when the patient expresses strong emotions of *fear*, *hatred* (anger, rage), *contempt* (hostility, disdain, degradation), or *romantic love* (sexualized feelings, or demands for succor, etc.). As applied to PTSD, the sequela of traumatic experiences involves those affects (fear, hatred, contempt, helplessness, love) that are prominent reactions to the stressors in the event. Trauma specific transference involves those strong emotions that the patient typically finds difficult to modulate. The patient then "transmits" his or her anxiety, defensiveness and fears to the therapist, often in an unconscious transmission, as a request for help because of the feelings of insecurity, uncertainty and confusion caused by the trauma experience. The therapist receives this anxiety-based transmission and attempts to "decode" its meaning while sustaining empathy in the treatment process.

Cohen (1952) lists 18 specific signs of anxiety and defensiveness in the analyst during treatment. These findings are particularly interesting for three basic reasons. First, though the publication is 50 years old, it is still relevant today to PTSD treatment approaches, although that was not Cohen's focus at the time. Second, it closely matches our description of Type I and Type II CTRs. Third, recent empirical research confirms the presence of all 18 signs of anxiety and defensiveness (Dalenberg, 2000; Danieli, 1988, 1994; Figley, 1995, 2002; Pearlman & Saatvikne, 1995; Wilson & Thomas, 1999). Figure 7.2 summarizes Cohen's (1952) analysis, and cross-indexes it with modes of empathic strain and Type I and Type II CTRs.

In 1991, Karen J. Maroda, after reviewing the psychoanalytic literature on countertransference, identified 21 signs, symptoms and behaviors associated with anxiety and defensiveness in therapists during the course of treatment. A study of Figure 7.3 reveals that Maroda's list of characteristics significantly overlaps Mabel B. Cohen's 1952 listing. Noteworthy in this group are indications of dysregulated affects, for example, arguing with the patient; atypical nervousness; overly critical behavior; persistent or transient states of anger, erotic, sexual and love affections towards and for the patient; feelings of being manipulated; and a range of withdrawal behaviors, such as canceling or forgetting sessions, and overly silent states. Further, subtle forms of dysregulated affects are evident in such actions as being overtly or covertly critical and judgmental, passively aggressive by repetition of rejected interpretations, and fears of being out of control.

As Figure 7.3 shows, the signs, symptoms and behaviors are about equally divided between Type I (avoidance) and Type II (overidentification) CTRs. All forms of empathic strain are evident, with empathic withdrawal and empathic enmeshment predominating. It is likely, however, that therapists will manifest alternating modalities of empathic strain. For example, awareness of empathic enmeshment (i.e., feeling "hooked," sexual feelings) may be compensated and defended against by empathic withdrawal or empathic repression. Similarly, feelings of guilt or impropriety from arguing with the patient, or being overly critical or judgmental, may be defended against by being overly silent and reserved.

There are many possibilities as to reactions and counterreactions to empathic strain during the treatment process. The strong convergence between Mabel Blake Cohen's analysis in 1952 and Karen J. Maroda's over 50 years later is impressive, as is the convergence on the manner in which these same signs, symptoms and behaviors are distributed across modalities of empathic strain and Type I and Type II countertransference processes.

Countertransference Reactions Among Professional Society Members (ISTSS, ISSD)

In the 1990s, Wilson and Lindy (1994), in their roles as organizational president, informally surveyed members of the International Society for Traumatic Stress Studies (ISTSS) on factors that indicated concern with countertransference in working with trauma clients and PTSD. Figure 7.4 summarizes these findings which were grouped into four categories: (1) physiological and physical reactions; (2) affective reactions; (3) psychological reactions; and (4) behavioral symptoms. This codification of symptoms is congruent with Cohen's (1952), Maroda's (1991) and Danieli's (1988) empirical research on CTRs among psychotherapists who work with Holocaust survivors.

Countertransference towards Holocaust Survivors

In the summary of her major findings, Danieli (1994) listed three areas of focus:

> ...(1) *various modes of defenses* which included numbing, denial, avoidance, distancing, clinging to professional roles, reduction to method and or theory; (2) *affective reactions* such as bystander's guilt, rage, with it variety of objects; dread and horror; shame and related emotions (e.g., disgust and loathing); grief and mourning; "me too; " sense of bond; privileged voyeurism; (3) *specific relational context* issues such as parent–child relationships; victim/liberator; viewing the survivor as a hero; and attention to attitudes towards Jewish identity. (p. 369, italics ours)

Danieli's (1988, 1994) research findings point to the tripartite interrelationship between *dysregulated affects* experienced during the treatment of Holocaust survivors: *affective reactions* (e.g., rage, guilt, shame, disgust, horror); *ego-defenses* related to emotional reactions by the therapist (e.g., denial, numbing, avoidance); and *role enactments* into which the therapist was cast in the therapeutic dyad (i.e., relational context).

Countertransference Relating to Southeast Asian Refugees and Ethnic Cleansing

It is interesting to note that nearly identical findings to Danieli's were reported by J. David Kinsie (1994) in a study of psychiatrists working with Southeast Asian refugees who had been subjected to brutalization which included ethnic cleansing, torture, witnessing executions, starvation, beatings, and political upheaval resulting in a loss of culture. Kinsie (1994) reports that, in terms of affective reactions to working with traumatized refugees, feelings of sadness, anger, depression, horror and disgust were prevalent. Additionally, forms of reexperiencing of the patient's trauma stories were present, as were sleep disturbances. As a result of daily immersion in therapeutic trauma work, "a heightened sense of arousal (cf. hyperarousal) with irritability was manifest and carried over after leaving work"(p. 257). Kinsie found that the work itself led to a strong sense of a uniquely shared experience, excessive identification with the patient and increased feelings of personal vulnerability. As Kinsie commented,

> Life is no longer the same. If beatings, starvation, torture, and mass killing can happen to our patients, *they can happen to us*. There is an increased awareness of the dangers of hatred and brutality that lie behind the mask of civilization we all wear, a sense of *being more vulnerable to life's dangers*. (p. 257, italics ours)

Dalenberg's Study of Countertransference with Treatment-Seeking Clients

In one of the few empirical studies of countertransference in the treatment of trauma and PTSD, Constance J. Dalenberg (2000) conducted a study of 84 patients who were questioned about their experiences in treatment. Each patient was seeking treatment for trauma related symptoms. The questionnaire contained 50 items nested within 13 sections, and addressed such issues as therapist disclosure, therapist avoidance tendencies, professional boundaries, affects (shame, pride, anger, blame, dependency, sex) and communication failures. Eighty-three percent of the study participants stated that their therapist "addressed joint avoidance of the trauma material" (p. 82), whereas only 10% "stated it was never avoided" (p. 82).

Based on her results, Dalenberg suggests that the negative therapeutic effects of avoidance tendencies can be mitigated in a variety of ways, including jointly addressing concrete instances of avoidance between therapist and client. Dalenberg hints at the fact that both the therapist and the client experience powerfully dysregulated affects. She concludes that: "the *discomfort* of the therapist in *listening to trauma* might not be an active (or even unconscious) wish to avoid, but rather a manifestation of the *fear* of causing further client *distress*" (p. 84, italics ours). From our perspective, it could be said that the fear extends, as well, to the therapist's anxiety of experiencing even more distress in listening to the patient's trauma account.

A MODEL OF AFFECT DYSREGULATION, ANXIETY STATES, COPING AND DEFENSE IN POST-TRAUMATIC THERAPY

Our analysis of anxiety and defensiveness in post-traumatic therapies enables discussion of a new conceptual model of the mechanisms that link affect dysregulation, anxiety states, empathy, transference, countertransference and ego-defenses. Figure 7.5 illustrates the dynamics of these processes and their patterns of operation during the course of treatment. This model applies to therapeutic dyads and group modalities of psychotherapy.

Trauma Narratives and Dysregulated Affects in Client and Therapist

To begin, we recognize that trauma patients proffer a trauma narrative and history of attempts to cope with their psychological injuries. In the telling and uncovering of the trauma history, the patient experiences states of *affect dysregulation* which vary in frequency, intensity, duration, severity and periodicity. The states of affect dysregulation have direct and unmistakable impact on the therapist, even if such effects are disavowed, denied, distorted or remain inaccessible to conscious awareness. The impact of the patient results in *dysregulated affective states* which disrupt (at some critical moment) the therapist's capacity for calm and sustained empathic attunement.

The disruption in the flow of empathic attunement triggers states of arousal and anxiety which become difficult to modulate. The process of coping with unmodulated affective states then sets in motion different forms of empathic strain which counterbalance modes of empathic attunement and are subjectively experienced as states of disequilibrium. These states of disequilibrium vary in intensity from mild to extreme forms of hyperarousal (e.g., hypervigilance, irritability, proneness to dissociation, anger, increased autonomic nervous system arousal, problems of concentration and memory, etc.). In response to lived through anxiety and disequilibrium, the therapist attempts to process the client's trauma transference processes.

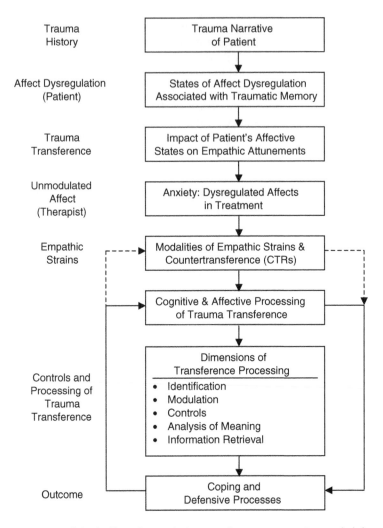

Figure 7.5 A model of affect dysregulation, anxiety states, coping and defense in post-traumatic therapy. Copyright John P. Wilson, 2003.

Dimensions of Transference Processing

We recognize five primary dimensions of transference processing: (1) identification of the patients *and* therapists affectively dysregulated states; (2) attempts to modulate the experienced disequilibrium and affect dysregulation; (3) utilization of control mechanisms in the service of affect modulation; (4) analysis of the meaning and clinical significance of trauma transference processes, including various role enactments into which the therapist can be cast; and (5) information retrieval from the seven channels of TSTT (see Figure 1.1). Thus, the cognitive and affective processing of the dual unfolding mechanisms and adaptive coping efforts is set in motion.

The model presented in Figure 7.5 is consistent with Allan N. Schore's conclusions on psychotherapy involving the primacy of dysregulated affective states caused by trauma. In discussing the role of defenses in treatment, Schore (2003b) states,

> A conception of *defense mechanisms as nonconscious strategies of emotional regulation for avoiding, minimizing, or converting affects that are too difficult to tolerate*, with an emphasis on dissociation and projective identification; these right brain defenses present the entrance into "dreaded states" charged with intense affects that can potentially traumatically disorganize the self-esteem. (p. 280, italics ours)

It would appear that the same defensive mechanisms are operative in therapists who treat traumatized patients suffering from PTSD and forms of self-pathologies (e.g., borderline states, narcissistic conditions, deinte-grated self-structures, identity diffusion, dissociative disorders, etc.). Understanding the dynamics of empathy is both critical and necessary for creating and facilitating a therapeutic alliance which labors to "recalibrate" dysregulated affects through positive allostatic tuning (see chapter 11 for a discussion). The term *sustained empathic attunement* is more than a descriptive phrase: it is a psychological precondition for effective treatment as well as a functioning psychobiological state of being.

REFERENCES

Cohen, M. B. (1952). Countertransference and anxiety. *Psychiatry, 15*, 231–243.

Cohen, M. B. (1988). Countertransference and anxiety. In B. Wolstein (Ed.), *Essential papers on countertransference* (pp. 64–84). New York: New York University Press.

Dalenberg, C. (2000). *Countertransference and PTSD*. Washington, DC: American Psychological Association Press.

Danieli, Y. (1988). Confronting the unimaginable: Psychotherapists' reactions to victims of the Nazi Holocaust. In J. P. Wilson, Z. Harel, & B. Kahana (Eds.), *Human adaptation to extreme stress* (pp. 219–237). New York: Plenum Press.

Danieli, Y. (1994). *Countertransference, trauma and training*. In J. P. Wilson & J. Lindy (Eds.), *Countertransference in the treatment of PTSD* (pp. 368–389). New York: Guilford Publications.

Erikson, E. H. (1968). *Identity, youth and crisis*. New York: Norton.

Figley, C. R. (1995). *Compassion fatigue*. New York: Brunner/Mazel.

Figley, C. R. (2002). *Treating compassion fatigue*. New York: Brunner-Routledge.

Hedges, L. (1992). *Interpreting the countertransference*. Northvale, NJ: Jason Aronson.

Kinsie, J. D. (1994). Countertransference in the treatment of Southeast Asian refugees. In J. P. Wilson & J. D. Lindy (Eds.), *Countertransference in the treatment of PTSD* (pp. 245–249). New York: Guilford Publications.

Kohut, H. (1977). *The restoration of the self*. New York: International Universities Press.

Lifton, R. J. (1967). *Death in life: The survivors of Hiroshima*. New York: Simon & Schuster.

Lifton, R. J. (1976). *The life of the self*. New York: Simon & Schuster.

Lifton, R. J. (1993). From Hiroshima to the Nazi doctors: The evolution of psychoformative approaches to understanding traumatic stress syndromes. In J. P. Wilson & B. Raphael (Eds.), *International handbook of traumatic stress syndromes* (pp. 11–25). New York: Plenum Press.

Maroda, K. J. (1991). *The power of countertransference*. New York: Wiley.

McCann, L. & Pearlman, L. (1990). *Psychological trauma and the adult survivor*. New York: Brunner/Mazel.

Pearlman, L. & Saakvitne, K. (1995). *Trauma and the therapist*. New York: Norton.

Racker, H. (1957). The meaning and uses of countertransference. *Psychoanalytic Quarterly, 26*, 303–357.

Schore, A. N. (2003a). *Affect dysregulation and disorders of the self*. New York: Norton.

Schore, A. N. (2003b). *Affect regulation and the repair of the self*. New York: Norton.

Tansey, M. J. & Burke, W. F. (1989). *Understanding countertransference*. Hillsdale, NJ: Erlbaum.

Wilson, J. P. (2003). *Empathic strain and post-traumatic therapy*. New York: Guilford Publications.

Wilson, J. P., Friedman, M. J. & Lindy, J. D. (2001). *Treating psychological trauma and PTSD*. New York: Guilford Publications.

Wilson, J. & Lindy, J. (1994). *Countertransference in the treatment of PTSD*. New York: Guilford Publications.

Wilson, J. P. & Thomas, R. (1999). *Empathic strain and counter-transference in the treatment of PTSD*. Paper presented at the 14th annual meeting of the International Society for Traumatic Stress Studies, Miami, FL.

Wolfe, E. (1990). *Treating the self*. New York: Guilford Publications.

Wolstein, B. (1988). *Essential paper on countertransference*. New York: New York University Press.

8

Empathy and Traumatoid States

In work with victims of trauma and PTSD, empathy takes center stage. In any human relationship, empathy embraces many of the highest qualities of human nature: compassion for others, authentic understanding and communication, openness to experience, respect for human dignity, and a willingness to reach out and help others in unselfish ways. In nearly all forms of psychotherapy, especially in "depth" therapies, empathy has been viewed as a capacity, skill and vehicle for reaching knowledge and understanding of the internal psychological processes of clients and those who seek help for difficult life experiences (Kohut, 1977; Nathan & Gorman, 1998; Pearlman & Saakvitne, 1995; Slatker, 1987; Wolfe, 1990).

This chapter introduces the concept of *traumatoid states*. Traumatoid states are "trauma-like" states which develop in therapists as a result of repeated exposure to trauma clients, and the responsibility of trying to help these clients in a professional role. Such states reflect stress-evoked changes in the therapist, and are the counterparts of prolonged stress response syndromes in clients with PTSD. Traumatoid states—comprising what has previously been described as compassion fatigue, vicarious traumatization and secondary traumatic stress syndrome—can be best characterized as occupationally related stress response syndromes (OSRS). As we will discuss, affect dysregulation and empathic identification play a pivotal role in the development of traumatoid states.

Understanding traumatoid states requires knowledge of the configurations of the patient's trauma experiences which get transferred during treatment. In this regard, there is a convergence of scientific opinion that in the treatment of PTSD, dissociative disorder and self-pathologies, the overarching goal is to assist patients in resolving the injurious aspects of their traumatic experiences and to heal from states of traumatization (Nathan & Gorman, 1998; Schore, 2003a, 2003b; van der Kolk, McFarlane, & Weisaeth, 1997; Wilson, Friedman, & Lindy, 2001). Recovery from states of traumatization means the ability to move towards optimal functioning. The restoring of meaning and wholeness to personality includes the capacity to integrate the traumatic experience into the self, and to accept the trauma as a part of the patient's life story, but do so without debilitating symptoms or residues that would limit the capacity for growth, change and self-actualization.

To achieve this therapeutic objective, there must be a strong sense of connectedness between therapist and patient. This state of connectedness implies a positive and mutual relationship of trust, understanding and willingness to find pathways to healing. Empathy, as we have discussed it, is a process that enables the establishment of mutuality and trust (Knox, 2003). It is the precondition for therapeutic alliance, empathic bonding, honesty in communication and disclosure of how trauma alters the patient's inner world of reality.

True empathy is like a three-dimensional holographic representation of the client's inner world, replete with sensory and emotional resonance. Empathy, as a capacity and process, enables a therapist to enter the various portals of entry into the inner sanctum of ego-space, the vault of the unconscious, the "file drawers" and "storage cabinets" of traumatic memories, and the realm of right-brain governed dysregulated affect (Schore, 2003a, 2003b). Moreover, empathic identification with the client underlies the capacity to establish strong therapeutic alliances and establishes the potential for stress-evoked traumatoid states.

The empathic therapist, with his capacity for sustaining empathic attunement with a traumatized patient, is like a symphony conductor directing an orchestra with all of its instruments, sections and musical splendor. The symphony conductor anticipates the musical score with its signature keys of movements, parts, crescendos, high and low notes, changes in tonal scales, transpositions, modulations and syncopations. The conductor demonstrates the ability to bring the music to life. It is no easy task, since the conductor, like the good therapist, must be able to read the full musical score for the entire orchestral ensemble at one time, to know the parts of the musical score that make up the entirety of the written composition. So too, the empathic therapist must be able to read the levels of traumatization scripted into the patient's life, must know how to explore them with sensitivity, grace and facility, and thus lead to a natural "flow" in the rhythm of post-traumatic recovery.

Empathy is subject to the forces of stress, time pressures and external factors that impinge on its quality. Empathic strains involve factors that limit empathy and the processes of empathic attunement in which there is a loss of resonance, phasic synchrony, and congruence in communication. Empathic strains can be generated by aspects of the therapist (e.g., inexperience, prior history of personal trauma, etc.) or the patient (e.g., intensity of the trauma story; nature, cause and severity of injuries, etc.). These internal or external factors associated with empathic strain can also be conceptualized as allostatic changes which alter homeostatic conditions of "even-keeled," "smoothly flowing" forms of empathic functioning.

As applied to the understanding of empathic strain, allostatic load refers to excessive, continuous or repeated exposure to the client's state of traumatization, where the levels of intensity, severity and potential are high enough to evoke fear, helplessness, affect dysregulation, and pose challenges to systems of meaning, belief and ideology. In this regard, allostatic load occurs in both clients and therapists in a similar manner. In essence, this is the nature of trauma work in general, and post-traumatic therapies, in particular.

Empathic strains are omnipresent, ambiguous and inescapable. Stress overload, however, may result in the formation of traumatoid states. The larger question now arises as to how best to conceptualize, understand and manage the inevitable stresses of trauma work which present challenges to the effective use of empathy in treatment. How doe we fundamentally understand the consequences of dysregulated affects, empathic strain and the variety of psychological events that emanate from them, including countertransference, compassion fatigue, vicarious traumatization, secondary traumatic stress, somatization, changes in identity, values and spirituality?

THE NATURE OF TRAUMA WORK, POST-TRAUMATIC THERAPIES AND TREATMENTS

Figure 8.1 presents a conceptual paradigm for understanding the relationship of empathy to trauma work and post-traumatic treatment approaches. We will examine the nature of how empathy and empathic strains are associated with dysregulated affective states which, in turn, lead to three distinct and separate response patterns. These response patterns have been referred to as compassion fatigue (CF), secondary traumatic stress (STS) and vicarious traumatization (VT) (Figley, 1995, 2002; Pearlman & Saakvitne, 1995). We will now discuss the similarities and differences in these terms, and then show how they are correlated with professional and personal outcomes which include: (1) stress related syndromes (CF, STS, VT); (2) existential search for meaning; (3) countertransference; (4) somatization; (5) changes in identity and self-processes; (6) interpersonal relations; and (7) spirituality.

In order to facilitate clarity in our deliberations on how empathy relates to stress response syndromes connected with empathic strain and dysregulated affects, we will begin by discussing similarities and differences in terminology.

COMPASSION FATIGUE, SECONDARY TRAUMATIC STRESS AND VICARIOUS TRAUMATIZATION: THE NEED FOR DEFINITIONAL CLARITY

Figure 8.2 presents definitions of CF, STS, VT, secondary traumatic stress order (STSD), empathy, empathic strain and empathic attunement. Since empathy is a process central to understanding the stresses that impact its operation in psychotherapy and other work related to trauma victims, it is important to establish clarity in the definitions of these terms as well as their similarities and differences as constructs. As indicated in Figure 8.1, it is possible and meaningful to distinguish between these constructs which have theoretical significance for understanding stress response syndromes and their subsyndromes.

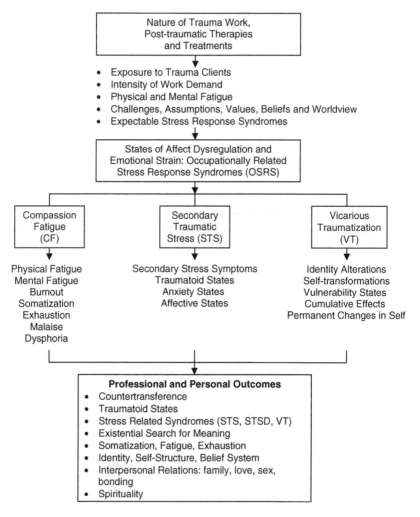

Figure 8.1 Trauma work, affect dysregulation and traumatoid states. Copyright John P. Wilson, 2003.

Empathy – "The psychobiological capacity to experience another person's state of being and phenomenological perspective at any given moment in time" (Wilson & Lindy, 1994)

Empathic Attunement – The psychobiological capacity to experience, understand and communicate knowledge of the internal psychological state of being of another person; empathic attunement is characterized by accurate emotional resonance, synchrony, the ability to decode multichanneled signal transmissions (e.g., nonverbal, emotional, physical/somatic states, cognitive processes, ego-defenses, ego-states, etc.) from another person, and manifest coetaneous matching responses experienced by recipient as being understood, "in phase" and "on target" with what they were sending as communications of information about their psychological processes (Wilson, 2003)

Empathic Strain – Interpersonal or other factors significantly affecting capacity for sustained empathic attunement and resulting in loss of capacity for resonance, synchrony, congruence in communication with stress; in psychotherapy and work with trauma patients, empathic strain refers to factors in the therapist, patient or in dyadic interaction that impair, limit or adversely impact the therapeutic process (Wilson, 2003)

Compassion Fatigue – A term that "can be used interchangeably by those who feel uncomfortable with STS and STSD" (Figley,1995); compassion fatigue is the stress and strain of caring for others who are ill or suffering due to medical illness or psychological maladies

Secondary Traumatic Stress (STS) – "The natural consequent behaviors and emotions resulting from knowing about a traumatizing event experienced by a significant other – the stress resulting from helping or wanting to help a traumatized or suffering person" (Figley, 1995)

Secondary Traumatic Stress Disorder (STSD) – "STSD is a syndrome of symptoms nearly identical to PTSD, except that exposure to knowledge about a traumatizing event experienced by a significant other is associated with a set of STSD symptoms, and PTSD symptoms are directly connected to the sufferer, the person suffering from primary traumatic stress" (Figley, 1995)

Vicarious Traumatization (VT) – "Vicarious traumatization refers to a transformation in the therapist's (or other trauma worker's) inner experience resulting from empathic engagement with the client's trauma material. That is, through exposure to clients' graphic accounts of sexual abuse experiences and to the realities of people's intentional cruelty to one another, and through the inevitable re-enactments in the therapy relationship, the therapist is vulnerable through his or her empathic openness to the emotional and spiritual effects of vicarious traumatization. These effects are cumulative and permanent, and evident in a therapist's professional and personal life"(1995)

Figure 8.2 Empathy and its relation to compassion fatigue, vicarious traumatization and secondary traumatization: The need for definitional clarity. Copyright John P. Wilson, 2003.

Compassion Fatigue

To begin, it is instructive to note that CF, in its simplest form, refers to the stress, strain and weariness of caring for others who are suffering from a medical illness or a psychological problem. Semantically, CF denotes lack of strength, languor, sluggishness, exhaustion, and loss of vigor, vitality and energy. One could say that a person experiencing CF is tired of helping and being compassionate.

Secondary Traumatic Stress

Secondary traumatic stress (STS) and secondary traumatic stress disorder (STSD) are conceptually linked to exposure to and involvement with those who have endured a traumatic event. As stated by Figley (1995), STS is "nearly the identical to PTSD," except that, instead of being directly involved with the precipitating traumatic event, the therapist or other professional is one step removed. In this sense, the helping professional gets exposed to the "wake" of trauma with its various ripple effects. By exposure to the traumatized person, the helper *indirectly* experiences some of the emotional injuries that are endured by the afflicted person. However, the definition of STS implies that the helper, through the process of empathy, can understand the nature and extent of the traumatic injuries to the person—to see and feel things from the latter's perspective.

Secondary traumatic stress disorder (STSD) is subsequently defined as a disorder "nearly identical to" PTSD, in which there develops acute, chronic or prolonged stress reactions which adversely impact psychological functioning. Figley (2002, p. 5) defines the disordered consequence of STS as a clinically significant impairment, as evidenced by "increased work conflict, missed work, insensitivity to clients, lingering distress caused by trauma material, reduced social support and poor stress coping methods." We prefer to refer to this syndrome as *traumatioid states* which include PTSD-like symptoms emanating from dysregulated affects and anxiety states in the helper (see chapter 10 for a complete discussion.)

Vicarious Traumatization

Vicarious traumatization (VT) differs significantly from the concepts of empathic strain, compassion fatigue and secondary traumatization (see Figure 8.2) because of its emphasis on "*transformation* in the therapist's (or other trauma workers) *inner experience* resulting from empathic engagement with client's trauma material" (p. 151, italics ours). Further, Pearlman and Saakvitne (1995) state that "the effects are *cumulative and permanent* and evident in both the therapist's professional and personal life" (p. 151, italics ours). The concept of VT involves transformative qualities relating to areas of the helper's "inner experience" which includes self-process, identity and systems of meaning and value. Indeed, Pearlman and Saakvitne rely on the constructivist self-development theory (CSDT) in their work on vicarious traumatization, and define self-capacities as

> inner experiences that allow the individual to maintain a consistent, coherent sense of identity, connection, and positive self-esteem ... [which includes] (1) the ability to tolerate strong affect and to integrate various affective experiences, (2) the ability to maintain a positive sense of self, and (3) the ability to maintain an inner sense of connection with others (1995, p. 69).

Vicarious traumatization, then, implies that basic self-capacities in terms of affect regulation, the structure of the self, and the nature of interpersonal connectedness can be transformed. Transformation processes themselves may take different forms, ranging from traumatoid states to altered systems of meaning, values and beliefs. In this regard, Pearlman and Saakvitne (1995) have gone beyond Figley's (1995, 2002) definition of CF, STS and STSD to suggest that the impact of exposure to patients suffering from trauma and PTSD extends to basic psychoformative processes, a point made by Robert J. Lifton (1976) in his book, *The Life of the Self*. In his various writings, Lifton has proposed that the effects of traumatization include basic changes in the subparadigms of psychoformative processes which he labeled *separation vs. connection, stasis vs. growth*, and *integration vs. disintegration* (Lifton, 1967, 1976, 1979, 1993).

A trauma may cause a survivor to feel isolated, separate and detached from his own inner processes of feeling, thinking and creating; to experience a cessation in personal growth (arrestation) and vision of the self-in-the-future; and to feel disintegrated as a coherent personality with a continuity in ego-identity. Pearlman and Saakvitne's (1995) concept of VT is similar to Lifton's subparadigms of psychoformative processes, since these concepts of "inner experience" may be impacted by exposure to the patient's state of traumatization and lead, in turn, to alterations in self-capacities. Pearlman and Saakvitne suggest that such effects to self-capacities may be *"cumulative and permanent"* rather than transient, acute or capable of "switching off" when involvement with the trauma client terminates.

Understanding the similarities and differences between the concepts of CF, STS and VT enables a broader view of these processes in work with trauma victims and PTSD. Figure 8.1 illustrates how these reactive processes are associated with exposure to trauma patients, and the resultant professional and personal outcomes.

NATURE OF TRAUMA WORK AND TRAUMATOID STATES

The nature of trauma work and psychotherapy with PTSD patients has five basic components: (1) exposure to traumatized clients and their injuries, dysregulated affective states and altered self-capacities; (2) task demands of daily work which usually involve intense encounters with patients; (3) physical and mental fatigue states; (4) challenges to assumptions, values, beliefs and world views; and (5) expectable stress response syndromes. These five factors, which are indigenous to work with trauma patients, directly influence the therapist's capacity to effectively manage them. As a consequence, states of affect dysregulaton and empathic strains are set in motion, influencing a wide range of intrapsychic and coping processes in the therapist. In a generic sense, we can refer to these reactions as *occupationally related stress response syndromes* (OSRS) which characterize the allostatic processes evoked by repetitive exposure to traumatized clients (see Wilson, Friedman, & Lindy, 2001, for a discussion). The allostatic loads of post-traumatic therapy, in turn, may lead to CF, STS, STSD and VT, as distinct but interrelated occupational stress response patterns.

Traumatoid States: Similarities and Differences in Occupational Stress Response Syndrome

What makes trauma work unique is that prolonged and repetitive exposure to clients creates an OSRS that is traumatoid in nature. In that sense, aspects of the client's injuries are absorbed emotionally by the helper. In capsule form, CF is characterized by physical and mental fatigue, malaise, exhaustion, and dysphoria; STS is *traumatoid* in nature, involving states of anxiety, secondary PTSD-like symptoms and dysregulated affects; VT impacts inner psychic states and self-capacities, altering them and producing permanent changes in self-functions, ego-states and systems of meaning.

The results of these processes (CF, STS, STSD, VT) have professional and personal consequences. Looking at the outcome processes of OSRS from a "crow's nest" perspective, we can see that they involve various forms of countertransference, traumatoid states, existential search for meaning and purpose, somatization, changes in identity, self-structure and belief systems, impacts to affiliative patterns of nurturance, love, family relations, sexuality and spiritual orientation.

It is important to understand the nature of personal and professional changes connected with exposure to trauma and PTSD patients in terms of therapist self-care, education, training and ethics. Chapter 11 addresses some of these issues and the more encompassing question of how optimal states of empathic functioning can be achieved and protected by "trauma membranes" (Lindy, 1989) which serve to support self-capacities for sustained empathic attunement.

EMPATHIC IDENTIFICATION, TRAUMATOID STATES AND OCCUPATIONALLY RELATED STRESS SYNDROMES

We can summarize the distinction between the processes of CF, STS and VT by showing their linkages to empathy and empathic strain.

Figure 8.3 illustrates that empathic strains emanate from the work of post-traumatic therapy or similar forms of occupational work with victims of trauma. The process of working with trauma patients is directly related to *empathic identification* in which the therapist or helping professional identifies with the pain and suffering of clients and their efforts to recover from the traumatic events they have endured. Through the process of *empathic identification* arises the potential for CF, STS and VT which are distinct but interrelated psychological processes. Respectively, then, CF concerns the fatigue of caring; STS refers to the acquisition of traumatoid states; and VT specifies cumulative and permanent transformations in self-capacities. These three forms of response to trauma work comprise OSRS, each with its own unique characteristics, which impact a wide range of personal and professional areas of coping and adaptation.

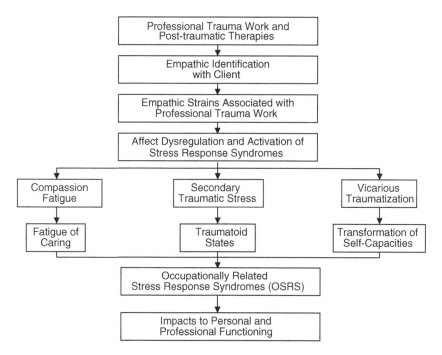

Figure 8.3 Empathic identification and empathic strain in the development of occupationally related stress response syndromes. Copyright John P. Wilson, 2003.

REFERENCES

Figley, C. (1995). *Compassion fatigue*. New York: Brunner/Mazel.

Figley, C. (2002). *Treating compassion fatigue*. New York: Brunner-Routledge.

Friedman, M. J. (2000a). *Posttraumatic and acute stress disorders*. Kansas City, MO: Compact Clinicals.

Friedman, M. J. (2000b). *Post-traumatic stress disorder: The latest assessment and treatment strategies*. Kansas City, MO: Compact Clinicals.

Knox, J. (2003). Trauma and defenses: Their roots in relationship: An overview. *Journal of Analytical Psychology, 48*, 207–233.

Kohut, H. (1977). *The restoration of the self*. New York: International Universities Press.

LeDoux, J. E. (1996). *The emotional brain*. New York: Simon & Schuster.

Lifton, R. J. (1967). *Death in life: The survivors of Hiroshima*. New York: Simon & Schuster.

Lifton, R. J. (1976). *The life of the self*. New York: Simon & Schuster.

Lifton, R. J. (1979). *The broken connection: On death and the continuity of life*. New York: Basic Books.

Lifton, R. J. (1993). From Hiroshima to the Nazi doctors: The evolution of psychoformative approaches to understanding traumatic stress syndromes. In J. P. Wilson & B. Raphael (Eds.), *International handbook of traumatic stress syndromes* (pp. 11–25). New York: Plenum Press.

Lindy, J. D. (1989) Transference and posttraumatic stress disorder. *Journal of the American Academy of Psychoanalysts, 17*(3), 397–413.

McEwen, B. (1998). Protective and damaging effects of stress mediators. *Seminars of the Beth Israel Deaconess Medical Center, 338*(3), 171–179.

Nathan, P. E. & Gorman, J. M. (1998). *Treatments that work*. New York: Oxford University Press.

Pearlman, L. & Saakvitne, K. (1995). *Trauma and the therapist*. New York: Norton.

Schore, A. N. (2003a). *Affect dysregulation and repair of the self*. New York: Norton.

Schore, A. N. (2003b). *Affect regulation and the repair of the self*. New York: Norton.

Slatker, E. (1987). *Countertransference*. Northvale, NJ: Jason Aronson.

van der Kolk, B., McFarlane, A. C. & Weisaeth, L. (1997). *Traumatic stress*. New York: Guilford Publications.

Wilson, J. P., Friedman, M. J. & Lindy, J. D. (2001). *Treating psychological trauma and PTSD*. New York: Guilford Publications.

Wilson, J. & Lindy, J. (1994). *Countertransference in the treatment of PTSD*. New York: Guilford Publications.

Wolfe, E. (1990). *Treating the self*. New York: Guilford Publications.

9

Therapist Reactions in Post-Traumatic Therapy: A Study of Empathic Strain in Trauma Work

This chapter describes an empirical study of clinicians' reactions to working with trauma victims. The study is designed to address several basic questions with regard to trauma work, psychotherapy and counseling of clients suffering from trauma-related psychological problems such as PTSD, dissociative disorders and their allied conditions (e.g., major depression, generalized anxiety disorder and substance abuse). The attempt is to understand the types of empathic strains, CTRs, symptoms of compassion fatigue, secondary traumatic states and vicarious traumatization that clinicians may have experienced in the course of their professional work. The purpose is to ascertain whether or not the history of the therapists, in terms of abuse and trauma, is associated with different types of empathic strains and countertransference, and the trauma clientele that they chose to work with in a professional role; and further, whether or not doing trauma work, primarily psychotherapy, social work and counseling, had an impact on personal values and relationships, worldview and beliefs about the nature of humankind and the meaning of life.

With the aim of learning, to the extent possible, through questionnaire data and open-ended questions, whether or not these professionals reported the onset of symptoms and changes in behavior that were due to repeated exposure to traumatized clients, our study seeks the answers to several issues on empathic strain: Did the participants develop symptoms, reaction tendencies and behaviors similar to those of their clients? Does working with traumatized clients produce sufficient stress to lead to significant levels of empathic strain in therapists? If so, in what ways are therapists impacted by their work with traumatized clients, and are there discernible and distinctive patterns of reactions that vary among them? Are there different reactive styles of therapists to traumatized clients suffering from trauma-related psychiatric and psychological disorders such as PTSD, dissociative disorders, self-pathologies and changes in the trajectory of personality development across the life cycle? Do the therapists report empathic strains and Type I and Type II CTRs? Do they have difficulty in maintaining professional boundaries and disclosing their CTRs to supervisors, colleagues and partners?

THEORETICAL AND CONCEPTUAL FRAMEWORK OF THIS STUDY

The study primarily utilized Wilson and Lindy's (1994) conceptual framework of modalities, empathic strain and Type I and Type II CTRs to guide construction of the Clinicians' Trauma Reaction Survey (CTRS) questionnaire during the mid-1990s. Additionally, the work on vicarious traumatization (McCann & Pearlman, 1990; Pearlman & Saakvitne, 1995) and compassion fatigue (Figley, 1995) was used to assist in the construction of items that would assess the dimensions of secondary stress reactions. A review of the psychoanalytic literature on countertransference was undertaken to identify signs, symptoms and behavioral indices suggestive of empathic strain, loss of empathic attunement, and CTRs and their manifestation in the treatment process (Thomas, 1998).

DEVELOPMENT OF THE CLINICIANS' TRAUMA REACTION SURVEY

Item categories for the Clinicians' Trauma Reaction Survey (CTRS) were developed in order to operationalize the constructs of empathic strain (four modalities) and countertransference (two typologies), as detailed by Wilson and Lindy (1994) in their book, *Countertransference in the Treatment of PTSD*. As noted in chapter 5, Type I CTRs (avoidance, counterphobia, detachment) have two corresponding modalities of empathic strain, reflective of the therapist's struggle to maintain good empathic attunement while working with trauma clients: *Empathic Withdrawal* (EW); and *Empathic Repression* (ER). Type II CTRs also have two modalities of empathic strain: *Empathic Disequilibrium* (ED); and *Empathic Enmeshment* (EN).

The items developed for the CTRS were designed to assess reactions of attendant professionals in several areas: (1) unmodulated affects to the trauma narratives of patients; (2) somatic complaints (e.g., headaches); (3) symptoms of PTSD classified according to the DSM-IV diagnostic criteria; (4) impacts to personal beliefs, values, relationships, worldview and self-functioning (i.e., identity, sense of meaning and purpose, etc.); and (5) DSM-IV associative features for PTSD, acute distress disorder, depression and anxiety. The CTRS is contained in the Appendix.

FACE AND CONTENT VALIDITY: AN ITERATIVE PROCESS

The CTRS was developed in 1996, and pilot tested for the next year with various professional groups who attended seminars, workshops and educational courses (e.g., Harvard Medical School; Harding Psychiatric Hospital). The pilot test respondents, all traumatic stress specialists, were interviewed about the instrument and their reactions to completing it. Based on interviews and written comments about their reactions, the CTR items were rewritten, discarded or added to the questionnaire. For example, a noted expert suggested adding an item (item 95) on experiencing "an adrenaline rush or high" while working with trauma clients.

All the professionals in the pilot study affirmed the need for such an instrument, found it stimulating and valuable to complete, and observed that it generated reflections on the nature of their work with clients. Upon completion of the pilot phase of the study, a 100-item version was formatted; this version contained 17 demographic questions for obtaining information on gender, licensure, years of experience in trauma work, self-disclosure of professional/personal concerns, personal trauma history, trauma clientele, extent of education and training in PTSD, percentage of time spent with trauma clients on an average basis, and patients that they would refer to other professionals. The 100 items were scored on a five-point Likert scale of (0) *never,* (1) *rarely,* (2) *sometimes,* (3) *often,* (4) *always.*

In December 1996, a random mailing was sent to 1,000 members of the International Society for Traumatic Stress Studies (ISTSS) and the International Society for the Study of Dissociative Disorders (ISSD). The sample, obtained with the support and endorsement of both professional societies, was computer generated and sent to members possessing designation of clinical work with trauma clients and *at least two years of professional membership.* A return sample of $N=345$ (34.5%) was received during the first six months of 1997 and was used for statistical analysis (Thomas, 1998).

Statistical Analyses

The Appendix contains the CTRS. Internal consistency of the items was .95 as measured by Cronbach's alpha test. Statistical analyses included measures of central tendency (e.g., percentage of respondents endorsing each item), bivariate correlations and factor analysis. An Oblimin Rotation, which assumes interrelationship between the derived factors, was selected as the factor analysis procedure. A Varimax Rotation, which assumes orthogonality among the factors, was also employed and yielded similar dimensions as the Oblimin Rotation, but with less stability among the factors.

FACTOR ANALYSIS OF DATA FROM CLINICIANS' TRAUMA REACTION SURVEY

Figures 9.1–9.5 present the results of the five-factor Oblimin solution which accounted for 42.9% of the overall scale variance.

Items comprising the five factors showed high internal consistency. Cronbach's alpha ranged from .92 to .75. Across the five factors, item loadings ranged from .80 to −.65. Some items are negatively correlated with specific factor clusters, since respondents rarely or never endorsed the item. The Oblimin solution showed moderate but significant correlations between each of the five factors (Thomas, 1998).

Select Sample Demographics

Analysis of data from the 345 responses to the CTRS showed approximately 70% of the sample to be middle-aged (46 years of age or older), some 60% of the respondents being female. Around 54% communicated personal traumatic experiences or abuse histories. As compared with the general population, a higher percentage of this sample identified themselves as atheists, or followers of a nonsecular spiritual orientation or members of an Eastern religion. About 66% reported holding a Ph.D. or M.D., and approximately 25% as holding multiple licenses. Around 25% of the respondents claimed to have between 15 and 20 years experience as mental health workers, while 41% stated that they had been career trauma workers for over 21 years, and as many as 70% that they had been working with traumatized clients for 10 or more years. Approximately 46% asserted that more than half their cases per year were trauma related, and 40% reported devoting more than 20 hours per week to work with traumatized clients. About 60% had training in PTSD and post-traumatic therapy through seminars, conferences, personal reading and literature reviews. Only 22.7% had professional education in trauma therapy in academic institutions.

Traumatized Populations Treated by the Sample

Traumatized client populations treated by this sample of attendant professionals included representatives of sexual abuse: emotional abuse: sexual assault; attempted suicide; battered spouse/significant other; medical trauma; violent crime victim; witness of violence; war veteran; severe personal injury; traumatic separation; sexual/gender

Item Loadings	Double Loadings	Item #	Item Description
.75		59	After meeting with my trauma clients I have found myself to be **hypervigilant** of what is happening around me.
.75		57	I have found myself to be **less trusting** of strangers since meeting with my trauma client(s).
.61		56	I have found myself **reacting as my trauma client(s) migh**t (e.g., exaggerated startle response, on edge in crowds...).
.59		87	In my professional work with trauma I have experienced **vicarious traumatization**.
.58		68	After being exposed to trauma stories I have experienced **more concern about the safety of those I hold dear.**
.57		63	After meeting with trauma client(s) I have **difficulty getting the image of their trauma story out of my mind.**
.56	Factor V −.34	33	I have found myself "**haunted**" by my client(s) and their trauma history.
.53		61	Due to the impact of my trauma client(s), I have found myself **reappraising my own beliefs and values.**
.52		69	After meeting with trauma clients I have experienced a sense that my **life could be short or shortened prematurely.**
.50		60	I have experienced **disillusionment** about the human condition due to work with trauma clients.
.50		72	After meeting with my trauma client(s) I have felt **overwhelmed that there is evil, abuse and victimization in the world.**
.48		3	I have experienced a sense of **personal vulnerability** listening to the trauma story of client(s).
.46		83	I have experienced **feelings of grief, mourning and sadness** during or after meeting with my trauma client(s).
.46	Factor III .46	79	Because of my work with trauma clients I have felt a **deepened sense of sadness** at what some people are capable of doing.
.45		34	I have had **strong emotional reactions** to my trauma client(s) which lasted well beyond our meeting.
.44		16	I have **wanted to exclude from my awareness the disturbing content** of my client's trauma story.
.44		82	Since working with trauma I have felt that **I am different now from how I was before I started the work.**

Figure 9.1 Oblimin rotated factor loadings for Factor I: Intrusive Preoccupation With Trauma.

.42	Factor III	70	I have experienced **frustration or anger that society** has not done more to prevent abuse and victimization.
	.36		
.40		76	After working with my trauma client(s) I have been **preoccupied with thoughts and feelings about trauma and abuse.**
.40	Factor IV	66	After meeting with my trauma client(s) I have experienced a **loss of interest in activities that I previously enjoyed.**
	.37		
.40		1	I have felt **overwhelmed by my client's trauma story**.
.37	Factor III	77	Due to my work with trauma clients I have experienced a **deepened search for meaning** as to why victimization occurs.
	.41		
.35	Factor III	89	I am **touched** by my trauma clients and their stories.
	.50		
.35		45	After meeting with my trauma client(s) I have experienced an **inability to fall asleep or stay asleep** through the night.
.34		41	I have been **so emotionally charged** from working with my trauma client(s) that it **seemed as if I were the victim too.**

Figure 9.1 (continued)

identification/orientation; occupational trauma; transport disaster; stalking; hijack; hostage; second generation Holocaust; natural disaster; Holocaust survivor; civilian war survivor; political/torture victim; refugee; and technological disaster.

Personal Trauma History and the Practice of Post-Traumatic Therapy

Of the 345 respondents, 186 (or 54%) of the sample indicated personal traumatic experiences or abuse histories. The top four categories of personal trauma reported are as follows: around 25%, personal experiences of emotional abuse as child or adult; some 18%, subjection to sexual abuse during childhood; about 14%, personal familiarity with medical trauma; and approximately 11%, personal experiences of physical abuse as child or adult. Females reported significantly more personal trauma history than did males (Thomas, 1998).

The respondents who recounted a personal chronicle of trauma had been treating clients with a similar type of traumatic experience. For example, 93% who reported an individual saga of emotional abuse,

Item Loadings	Double Loadings	Item #	Item Description
.73		9	Listening to my trauma client(s), I have found my **attention lapsing/my thoughts drifting.**
.68		8	While with my trauma client(s) I have found myself **thinking about things unrelated** to my clients and their issues.
.61		51	I have found myself **growing drowsy or sleepy** while listening to my trauma client(s).
.58		55	I have found it **difficult to concentrate** on my client's trauma story as it was being told.
.57		52	I have experienced myself **"numbing out"** while listening to my trauma client(s).
.52		78	I have experienced **difficulty remembering** all that my trauma clients have told me.
.52		24	I have experienced **emotional or empathic detachment** while working with trauma clients.
.42	Factor IV .34	84	In my work with trauma clients I have experienced being **"out of touch"** with my own emotions or feelings.
.41		44	During or after meeting with my trauma clients I have **experienced headaches.**
.41		12	I have **experienced unwanted feelings and memories from my past** while listening to my trauma client(s).
.40		6	Listening to my trauma client(s) I have felt a **need to hide behind a professional role.**
.38		50	I have experienced **somatic reactions** (e.g., bodily pain, throat constriction, muscle tension) during or after meetings with trauma client(s).
.37		62	I have found myself **"steering" the conversation** with trauma client(s) in the direction that **makes me feel the least distress.**
.36	Factor 4 .34	85	I have experienced a **loss a sensuality and emotional sensitivity** due to my immersion in trauma work.
.36		46	I have experienced **greater irritability and proneness to anger** after meeting with my trauma client.
.34		11	While listening to my trauma client(s) I have **thought about difficult emotional experiences in my own life.**
.34		53	I have experienced **changes in my breathing pattern** while listening to my clients' trauma stories.
.32	Factor V −.37	23	I have experienced the **wish that my trauma client does not show up for scheduled appointments.**
.31	Factor IV .50	67	I have felt a **need to be alone or isolated** from others after meeting with my trauma clients.

Figure 9.2 Oblimin rotated factor loadings for Factor II: Avoidance and Detachment.

Item Loadings	Double Loadings	Item #	Item Description
.70		36	I have experienced a **protective attitude** toward my trauma client(s).
.64		35	I have felt **a strong urge to solve the problems** of my trauma client(s).
.61		39	I have thought of my **client(s) as heroic** for enduring the traumatic experience.
.59		22	I have experienced a **need to protect, rescue or shelter** my trauma client(s) from the abuses they have suffered.
.53		17	I have experienced **concerns** for my trauma client(s) that **extend beyond the work setting.**
.52	Factor V .39	96	I have experienced a **heightened sense of meaning/reason** for being when I do this work
.50	Factor I .35	89	I am **touched** by my trauma clients and their stories.
.50		40	I have **done more** for my trauma client(s) **than is actually required by my profession.**
.50		37	I have **felt like a liberator or savior** in my helping role.
.49		20	I have experienced a **need to advocate** for my client(s) due to the victimization they endured.
.48	Factor V .34	95	I have **experienced an adrenaline rush or high** while working with trauma clients.
.46	Factor I .46	79	Because of my work with trauma clients I have felt a **deepened sense of sadness at what some people are capable of doing.**
.43	Factor V −.31	19	I have found it **difficult to maintain firm boundaries** with my trauma client(s) due to the intensity of their needs.
.41	Factor I .37	77	Due to my work with trauma clients I have **experienced a deepened search for meaning as to why victimization occurs.**
.36	Factor I .42	70	I have experienced **frustration or anger that society has not done more to prevent abuse.**
.36		71	I have had **thoughts of avenging the wrongs committed against my trauma client(s).**
.34		18	I have felt a strong **sense of personal identification** with some of my trauma clients.
−.32	Factor V −.45	100	**(Disagree that)** Due to the nature of my work with trauma clients I have secretly **wished** I were **doing** something else with my **career.**

Figure 9.3 Oblimin rotated factor loadings for Factor III: Over-Involvement and Identification.

Item Loadings	Double Loadings	Item #	Item Description
.81		73	I have **not felt safe or trusting enough of my colleagues** to be able to talk about my work and experience with trauma clients.
.76		75	I have felt a **lack of internal and/or external support** in my work with trauma survivors.
.73		74	Due to my work with trauma clients I have **felt alienated from others who do not understand the work.**
.71		91	I have **felt abandoned by my supervisors or colleagues** in issues with my trauma clients.
.65		90	I have been **reluctant to speak honestly to colleagues/supervisors for fear of being viewed as a novice, inept or wrong.**
.64		81	I have **felt I cannot burden others** with the traumatic events I have heard, so I keep them to myself and **deal with them alone.**
.54		80	I have found it **difficult to disclose information** to others about the horrific traumatic events I learn of through my work.
.50	Factor II .31	67	I have felt a **need to be alone or isolated** from others, after meeting with my trauma client(s).
.47		65	After meeting with trauma clients I experience **difficulty telling others about the emotional impact of the "work" I do.**
.37	Factor I .40	66	After meeting with my trauma clients I have experienced a **loss of interest in activities** that I previously enjoyed.
.34	Factor II .42	84	In my work with trauma clients I have experienced being **"out of touch" with my own emotions or feelings.**
.34	Factor II .36	85	I have experienced a **loss of sensuality and emotional sensitivity** due to my immersion in trauma work.
.34		48	I have experienced **more stress and tension** after meeting with my trauma clients.

Figure 9.4 Oblimin rotated factor loadings for Factor IV: Professional Alienation.

either during childhood or as adults, had treated trauma patients who were victims of an identical kind of abuse; about 90% who reported a personal narrative of childhood sexual abuse had been dealing with trauma clients who had endured the same type of abuse; an impressive 100% of the respondents who affirmed being war veterans had themselves been treating war veterans; as many as 92% of respondents reporting battery by a spouse had been caring for patients who were

Item Loadings	Double Loadings	Item #	Item Description
.39	Factor III .52	96	I have experienced a **heightened sense of meaning or reason for being** when I do trauma work.
.34	Factor III .48	95	I have experienced an **adrenaline rush or high** while working with trauma clients.
−.31	Factor III .43	19	**(Disagree that)** I have found it difficult to **maintain firm boundaries** with my trauma clients due to the intensity of their needs.
−.33		28	**(Disagree that)** I have experienced **thoughts of terminating therapy** even when I knew there was more work to be done.
−.33		13	**(Disagree that)** I have found myself not wanting to **believe my clients' trauma stories.**
−.34	Factor I .56	33	**(Disagree that)** I have found myself **"haunted"** with my clients and their trauma history.
−.35		31	**(Disagree that)** I have wished that **prescribed medications would make my trauma client easier** to work with.
−.37	Factor II .32	23	**(Disagree that)** I have experienced the **wish** that my trauma **clients not show up** for the scheduled appointments.
−.39		15	**(Disagree that)** I have become **frustrated** with trauma clients who are difficult to move forward.
−.45	Factor III −.23	100	**(Disagree that)** Due to the nature of my work with trauma clients I have secretly **wished I were doing something else with** my career.
−.46		14	**(Disagree that)** I have found myself **wondering why I chose to work with trauma clients.**
−.47		25	**(Disagree that)** I have had **thoughts of referring** my trauma clients to someone else for help.
−.50		2	**(Disagree that)** I have experienced **uncertainty as to my ability** to work with trauma clients.
−.65		26	**(Disagree that)** There have been times when I have **wished** that I did **not have to work with** my **trauma client(s).**

Figure 9.5 Oblimin rotated factor loadings for Factor V: Professional Role Satisfaction.

themselves battered spouses; around 89% of the sample indicating a history of physical abuse had been attending to clients who had sustained physical abuse; approximately 89% of the sample with a history of attempted suicide had been treating patients who had attempted suicide; and some 81% of the sample with a personal history of adult sexual assault reported treating clients who had suffered from the same kind of traumatic experience.

THERAPISTS' REACTIONS TO TRAUMA WORK: FIVE FACTORS REFLECTING EMPATHIC STRAIN AND TYPE I AND TYPE II COUNTERTRANSFERENCE

Factor I: Intrusive Preoccupation with the Nature of Trauma Work Experiences

Factor I consists of 25 items with item loadings between .75 and .34, a Cronbach's alpha of .92, eigenvalue of 16.9, and accounts for 22.5% of variance in the measure.

Factor I comprises CTRS items suggestive of reexperience phenomena. Reexperience reactions in therapists appear to parallel the reactions of traumatized clients on several levels: (1) psychological distress as evidenced by difficulty in removing traumatic images of clients' trauma stories; preoccupation with unwanted thoughts or feelings about trauma and abuse, strong emotional reactions, feeling "as if a victim, too," and loss of interest in previously enjoyed activities; (2) physiological distress as evidenced by hypervigilance, exaggerated startle response, edginess in crowds, inability to fall or stay asleep, and heightened states of arousal; (3) alterations in personal constructs, such as changes in worldview, self-identity, ways of being in the world, and systems of belief and meaning.

The items with the highest loadings on Factor I include:

- After meeting with my trauma client(s), I have found myself to be hypervigilant as to what is happening around me.
- Since meeting with my trauma client(s) I realize that I have become less trusting of strangers.
- I find that I react as my trauma client(s) might (e.g., exaggerated startle response, on edge in crowds ...).
- In my professional work with trauma, I have experienced vicarious traumatization.
- After being exposed to trauma stories, I have experienced more concern about the safety of those I hold dear.
- After meeting with trauma client(s), I have difficulty in getting the images of their trauma story out of my mind.
- I have discovered that I am "haunted" by my client(s) and their trauma history.
- Due to the impact of my trauma client(s), I have found myself reappraising my own beliefs and values.

Factor I indicates reactions such as intrusive images, irritability, autonomic nervous system arousal, and physiological reactions. As discussed by Wilson and Lindy (1994), conscious reliving by the therapist may be stimulated by exposure to clients' personal struggles to integrate their own traumatic experiences. Factor I also reveals that the therapist's beliefs, attitudes, values and symptoms of meaning are affected by the work and load on this factor. For example, 92.4% noted, "I am different now from how I was before I began working with trauma clients"; about 89.5% reported that they found themselves reappraising personal beliefs and values; around 82% related experiences of difficulty in getting client trauma images out of the mind; some 82.6% indicated experiences of disillusionment about the human condition due to work with trauma clients; and 45.2% reported experiences of loss of interest in activities previously enjoyed.

THEMATIC SCHEMAS AND TRAUMAS IMPACT ON THERAPISTS

The following are representative of CTRS respondents' open-ended comments pertaining to themes inherent in Factor I:

While I may not have felt these things always or often (overwhelmed that there is evil, abuse, and victimization in the world; difficulty getting the image of their trauma story out of my mind; heightened concern about the safety of those held dear), I have felt them very strongly. There was a period when dealing with the existential problems was what my life was mostly about. (Female, Ph.D., with over 15 years of experience working with trauma clients.)

I feel one develops a sense of personal vulnerability that predisposes [one] to seeing and expecting trauma (which I do not like). (Male, Ph.D., with over 15 years in the field, and over 10 years of experience with trauma clients.)

I believe that my long-term work with trauma has in fact substantially altered my interpersonal sphere—to the extent that it's symptomatic of a defense against what I'm exposed to regarding content and the impact of long-term involvement in relationships with traumatic transference ... (Female, CSW, with over 15 years of experience with trauma clients.)

I feel different since working extensively with trauma: torture, political repression, war—somewhat less "light" or spontaneous, a little quicker and deeper to anger. My views on humanity are very cynical and continue to evolve. (Male, Ph.D., with over 10 years in the field, and over 5 years of experience with trauma clients.)

Since I have been working for 20 years with trauma survivors [these] answers are different from what they would have been sometime ago. Also, I am burned out as you can see from all I have heard, and recently it has dawned on me that my self and worldview has significantly changed from doing the work. I am in the process of reclaiming my life and not be so immersed in trauma stories. Also, I doubt the effect of psychotherapy as a change format. It's made me look at myself as a human being, where I am on the continuum of victim–perpetrator–observer/denial. How can I live with what I know? I am currently working on being a thriver, not just survivor with my clients. (Female, LICSW, with over 21 years in the field, and over 15 years of experience with trauma clients.)

Factor II: Avoidance and Detachment

Factor II consists of 19 items with items loadings between .73 and .31, a Cronbach's alpha of .87, eigenvalue of 4.5, and accounts for 6.0% of the variance.

Factor 2 consists of item loadings characterizing avoidance and detachment reactions. These reactions include loss of attention, distraction, sleepiness, problems of concentration, emotional numbing, memory problems, feeling "out of touch," and somatic complaints (e.g., headaches). Other avoidance and detachment responses comprise overreliance on technique, directed "steering" of the client's conversation, preoccupation with personal matters, and a wish that clients would not show up for scheduled appointments. Items loading on these factors are desires to be alone or isolated after meeting with trauma clients.

The items with the highest loadings on Factor II include:

- While listening to my trauma client(s), I have noticed my attention lapsing/my thoughts drifting.
- While with my trauma client(s), I have found myself thinking about things unrelated to my clients and their issues.
- I have observed myself growing drowsy or sleepy while listening to my trauma client(s).
- I have found it difficult to concentrate on my client(s) trauma story as it was being told.
- I have felt myself "numbing out" while listening to my trauma client(s).
- I have experienced difficulty in remembering all that my trauma client(s) have told me.
- I have experienced emotional or empathic detachment while working with trauma clients.

The following are representative of CTRS respondents' comments pertaining to themes inherent in Factor II:

I am concerned about not becoming calloused and indifferent, or turning off my emotional reactions to [clients'] abuse narratives. (Male, Ph.D., with over 21 years in the field, and over 6 years of experience with trauma clients.)

Made me think—I realize how "privately" numb I am during and after sessions. (Female, LICSW, with over 20 years in the field, and 10 years of working with trauma clients.)

Factor III: Overinvolvement and Identification

Factor III consists of 18 items with items loadings between .70 and −.32, a Cronbach's alpha of .87, eigenvalue of 3.5, and accounts for 4.7% of the variance.

The items loading on this factor reflect intensive involvement with trauma clients ranging from experiencing "an adrenaline rush" to protective attitudes and personal advocacy on behalf of clients' welfare. Respondents report viewing their clients as heroic, and experience concerns for them that extend beyond the office, feeling compelled to be advocates, liberators or saviors. Items reflecting a sense of meaning from the work load here as to concerns with victimization and injustice in the world. A clear sense of personal identification with clients is also reflected in pro-social advocacy, a desire to avenge wrongs, and anger at society for allowing victimization to occur.

The items with the highest loadings on Factor III include:

- I have experienced a protective attitude toward my trauma client(s).
- I have felt a strong urge to solve the problems of my trauma client(s).
- I have thought of my client(s) as heroic for enduring the traumatic experience.
- I have experienced a need to protect, rescue, or shelter my trauma client(s) from the abuses they have suffered.
- I have endured concerns for my trauma client(s) that extend beyond the work setting.
- I have realized a heightened sense of meaning/reason for being when I do this work.
- I am touched by my trauma clients and their stories.
- I have done more for my trauma client(s) than is actually required by my profession.
- I have felt like a liberator or savior in my helping role.

Factor IV: Professional Alienation

Factor IV consists of 13 items with items loadings between .81 and .34, a Cronbach's alpha of .88, eigenvalue of 3.0, and accounts for 4.0% of the variance.

Factor IV reflects concerns with professional alienation, mistrust of colleagues and supervisors and a sense of isolation. This factor reveals a lack of perceived support for the work, reluctance to self-disclose, and "withdrawal" in the sense of losing interest in previously enjoyed activities. The sense of isolation and alienation also includes a reported loss of sensuality and emotional sensitivity. Additionally, this factor includes mistrust and increased states of tension.

The items with the highest loadings on Factor IV comprise

- I have not felt safe or trusting enough of my colleagues to be able to talk about my work and experience with trauma clients.
- I have felt a lack of internal and/or external support in my work with trauma survivors.
- Due to my work with trauma clients, I have felt alienated from others who do not understand the work.
- I have felt abandoned by my supervisors or colleagues in issues with my trauma clients.
- I have been reluctant to speak honestly to colleagues/supervisors for fear of being viewed as a novice, as inept or wrong.
- I have felt I cannot burden others with the traumatic events I have heard, so I keep them to myself and deal with them alone.
- I have found it difficult to disclose information to others about the horrific traumatic events I learn of through my work.
- I have felt a need to be alone or isolated from others, after meeting with my trauma client(s).

Factor IV (Professional Alienation) suggests that helping professionals are inhibited about disclosing work particulars to other professionals. They experience difficulty in discussing their therapeutic activities and the emotional impact of the work. Concerns related to self-disclosure were found in analyses of CTRS demographic item 11 (i.e., number of hours per month of peer counseling/supervision), and demographic item 13 (i.e., self-disclosure and sharing). The data indicated that

- 79.9% noted difficulty in disclosing aspects of their work
- 75% experienced alienation from others who did not understand the nature of their work
- 72.6% were aware of lack of internal or external support in their work with trauma clients
- 61.7% felt reluctance to speak honestly to colleagues or supervisors for fear of being viewed as a novice, or inept or wrong
- 58% felt abandoned by colleagues or supervisors in issues concerning their experiences with trauma clients.

Themes found in the items loading on Factor IV are similar to conflicts of actual trauma survivors who express shame, manifest estrangement and alienation, and fear misunderstanding, ridicule, judgment, blame and abandonment from the therapist they rely upon for help. Clients are often uncertain about disclosing the full trauma story for fear of being misunderstood, judged, held responsible for, not believed, or shamed by the events that they have experienced. A parallel theme is echoed in trauma therapist difficulties in self-disclosure to supervisors. In a similar way to the therapist's reaction to clients' case material, colleagues and supervisors may be confronted and confounded by their own resistance or CTR to the traumatic material brought to bear on by fellow professionals. They may simply lack understanding and empathy for the realities of this work and its potential for personal impact. Supervision, peer support, encouragement, consultation and collaboration provide a crucial service as a "trauma membrane" against the impact of vicarious exposure. The perceived lack of a protective membrane may leave the helping professional feeling isolated. Wilson and Lindy (1994) found incidents of supervisors of senior psychoanalysts unable to tolerate the content of trauma-related issues, and commented: "above all, this person could not hear me..." (p. XV).

When institutions fail to create an environment in which helping professionals feel part of a cooperative team, with shared values and a commitment to aid victims of trauma, the impact to the therapist is likely to be a negative one. This may create dual forms of countertransference and empathic stress reactions—one toward the institution, and one toward the client. Pearlman and Saakvitne (1995) point out that therapists in the field of PTSD and dissociation are caught in the middle of a "paradigm shift" which reflects controversies over terminology, techniques and constructs, as well as accreditation, funding and third party reimbursement. This fact can contribute to difficulties in maintaining dedication to the work.

Trauma professionals look to those doing the research and publishing for answers and support. One respondent commented,

> ...Other concerns center around the current controversy regarding recovered memories, dissociative disorders, ritual abuse, and organized mind control projects. I've been doing this work for 10 years, sought professional consultation, attended countless conferences and seminars, continue to read the latest literature and now, I'm supposed to throw out all this data and experience and client progress because it's unpopular to treat these clients and listen to them as we do all our other clients. (Female, MFCC, with over 10 years of working with trauma clients.)

Respondents to the CTRS remarked,

> Most of the colleagues I know who have worked with sexual abuse, ritual abuse, mind control programming, DID [dissociative identity disorder], etc., who are now between 40–50 years old (10 to 20 years in mental health) are wondering whether

it's worth it anymore, after this long, to have other professionals discount or "disbelieve" what they have seen in their offices on a daily basis for 10 to 20 years. It feels infuriating, isolating, abandoning, insulting, nonsupportive, etc. The work is too hard, complicated, painful and difficult to not feel. It's like telling an oncologist that cancer doesn't exist, or that he or she created it. I'll stop now. (Female, LICSW, with over 21 years in the field, and over 10 years of experience with trauma clients.)

[I have felt threatened or unsafe]—Absolutely—not because of my clients' threats toward me anymore, but the prejudice and even hatred of patients among some of my supervisors and colleagues. It's not safe to work in some places... I question whether I should consider the abuse I have sustained in the workplace due to being an "advocate" for PTSD patients as personal trauma history. (Male, M.D., with over 5 years of working with trauma clients.)

I wish you would include more about what feelings are aroused by fellow professionals. I spend about 20 hours a week in direct service to trauma victims (DID including a lot of ritual abuse), and I have been more traumatized by my clients' mistreatment in hospitals and psychiatry offices than I ever have been by the clients themselves. In my opinion, the field of mental health is truly in the Dark Ages when it comes to dealing with trauma—and managed care makes things worse. (No demographics given.)

I have felt abandoned by my supervisors or colleagues in issues with my trauma clients. I have not felt safe or trusting enough of my colleagues to be able to talk about my work and experience with trauma clients. My community is biomedical and denies PTSD and dissociation diagnosis. (Male, Ph.D., with over 20 years of working with trauma clients.)

Factor V: Professional Role Satisfaction

Factor V consists of 14 items, with item loadings between +.39 and −.65, a Cronbach's alpha of .75, eigenvalue of 2.3, and accounts for 3.0% of the variance. Of the items derived by Oblimin rotation loading on Factor V, most are negatively correlated. Note that the negative factor loadings are interpreted as the respondent disagreeing with the item as it appeared on the CTRS.

Factor V, entitled Professional Role Satisfaction, is characterized by positive attitudes toward work with traumatized populations. This factor suggests empathic equilibrium in the helping professional. The respondents look forward to working with trauma clients and are confident in their ability to do so. Frustrations with clients, and intrusive imagery or thoughts of trauma, are not experienced. Firm boundaries are maintained without difficulty. A sense of professional satisfaction, as well as a heightened sense of meaning or reason for being, is reported.

The items with the highest loadings on Factor V include

- (Respondents agreed to ...) I have experienced a heightened sense of meaning or reason for being when I do trauma work.
- (Respondents agreed to ...) I have experienced an adrenaline rush or high while working with trauma clients.
- (Respondents disagreed to ...) I have found it difficult to maintain firm boundaries with my trauma clients due to the intensity of their needs.
- (Respondents disagreed to ...) I have experienced thoughts of terminating therapy even when I knew there was more work to be done.
- (Respondents disagreed to ...) I have found myself not wanting to believe the trauma story of my clients.
- (Respondents disagreed to ...) I have found myself "haunted" with my clients and their trauma history.

Pearlman and Saakvitne (1995) note the rewards of doing trauma therapy, highlighting the dynamics of the transformation of the clients, the transformations of the therapist as professional, and the transformation of the therapist as person. Factor V is characterized by themes of increased professional satisfaction derived from the work. Respondents to the CTRS remarked,

> *After nearly 20 years in this work I have developed an unshakable faith in the courage, strength and ability to heal possessed by my clients. This allows me to maintain detached empathy without loss of my own feelings. I carry a strong sense of what is my burden to bear and what is theirs. By now, I have heard every kind of horror. I am now "unshakable." This does not mean I cannot appreciate their experience.* (Female, CMHC, with over 15 years of working with trauma clients.)

> *Twice [while completing the CTRS] I realized how my reactions have changed over the years. I trust myself so much more now, and know that I am a deeper, better person for the work I have done. At times I have been in awe of my clients' strengths. Sometimes trauma makes us a deeper, finer vessel. My work has also altered my own paradigms; I have more faith in the human psyche to survive.* (Female, LCSW, MFCC, with over 20 years of working with trauma clients.)

> *I think this work puts you most in touch with what it means to be fully human and all the pain, heartbreak, courage and healing that can be part of the human condition. This is not such a bad place.* (Male, Ph.D., with over 20 years in the field, and with over 10 years of working with trauma clients.)

> *Many of the changes I have experienced in working as a trauma therapist are positive changes—increased appreciation for the strength of the mind and its defenses, increased respect for children, deepened sense of connections to humanity and nature, more hope, more empathy.* (No demographics given.)

Answering these questions reminded me that the work I've done with trauma patients has been the most deeply satisfying work I've done, although I'm enjoying more "garden variety" work right now. I want to return (while continuing to balance my own needs and capacities) to trauma work as my major focus again, as I felt my talents were truly being used best when I did that kind of work. (Male, M.D., with 10 years experience in the field, and with over 5 years of working with trauma clients.)

The data from the factor analysis identified five distinct types of reactions to trauma work. These five factors correspond to Type I and Type II countertransference described by Wilson and Lindy's (1994) model and the four modalities of empathic strain: empathic disequilibrium, empathic enmeshment, empathic withdrawal and empathic repression. The results also indicate separate factor structures for professional satisfaction versus professional alienation. Chapter 10 covers a further discussion on the significance of these five factors as well as specific item endorsements as they pertain to the issues and validity of constructs, such as compassion fatigue, secondary traumatic stress reactions, vicarious traumatization and traumatoid states. However, the results of this study clearly indicate that there are different patterns of reactions to trauma work. These different "styles" of reaction to trauma work reflect personality, client and process variables which influence the tapestry of the therapeutic setting. Chapters 8 and 10 present a conceptual framework which encompasses these different dimensions and shows how they are related to empathy, affect dysregulation, stress response syndromes and the development of traumatoid states. As we will discuss further, traumatoid states are "PTSD-like" states which develop through repetitive and prolonged exposure to traumatized clients.

REFERENCES

Figley, C. R. (1995). *Compassion fatigue.* New York: Brunner/Mazel.

Figley, C. R. (2002). *Treating compassion fatigue.* New York: Brunner-Routledge.

Knox, J. (2003). Trauma and defenses: Their roots in relationship: An overview. *Journal of Analytical Psychology, 48,* 207–233.

Kohut, H. (1977). *The restoration of the self.* New York: International Universities Press.

LeDoux, J. E. (1996). *The emotional brain.* New York: Simon & Schuster.

Lifton, R. J. (1993). From Hiroshima to the Nazi doctors: The evolution of psychoformative approaches to understanding traumatic stress syndromes. In J. P. Wilson & B. Raphael (Eds.), *International handbook of traumatic stress syndromes* (pp. 11–25). New York: Plenum Press.

Lifton, R. J. (1967). *Death in life: The survivors of Hiroshima.* New York: Simon & Schuster.

Lifton, R. J. (1976). *The life of the self.* New York: Simon & Schuster.

Lifton, R. J. (1979). *The broken connection: On death and the continuity of life.* New York: Basic Books.

McCann, L. & Pearlman, L. (1990). *Psychological trauma and the adult survivor.* New York: Brunner/Mazel.

Nathan, P. E. & Gorman, J. M. (1998). *Treatments that work*. New York: Oxford University Press.

Pearlman, L. & Saakvitne, K. (1995). *Trauma and the therapist*. New York: Norton.

Schore, A. N. (2003a). *Affect dysregulation and repair of the self*. New York: Norton.

Schore, A. N. (2003b). *Affect regulation and the repair of the self*. New York: Norton.

Slakter, E. (1987). *Countertransference*. Northvale, NJ: Jason Aronson.

Thomas, R. B. (1998). *An investigation of empathic stress reactions among mental health professionals working with PTSD*. Unpublished doctoral dissertation, Union Institute, Cincinnati, OH.

van der Kolk, B., McFarlane, A. C. & Weisaeth, L. (1997). *Traumatic stress*. New York: Guilford Publications.

Wilson, J. P. (2004). PTSD and complex PTSD: Symptoms, syndromes and diagnoses. In J. P. Wilson & T. M. Keane (Eds.), *Assessing psychological trauma and PTSD* (2nd ed., pp. 1–47). New York: Guilford Publications.

Wilson, J. P., Friedman, M. J. & Lindy, J. D. (2001). *Treating psychological trauma and PTSD*. New York: Guilford Publications.

Wilson, J. & Lindy, J. (1994). *Countertransference in the treatment of PTSD*. New York: Guilford Publications.

Wolfe, E. (1990). *Treating the self*. New York: Guilford Publications.

10
Understanding the Nature of Traumatoid States

The concept of traumatoid states resulting from exposure to and intensive work with victims of trauma is a new conceptual development in the area of traumatology. At present, we have only a few empirical studies of compassion fatigue, secondary traumatic stress, vicarious traumatization, and countertransference (Figley, 1995, 2002; Dalenberg, 2000; Thomas, 1998). The results of these studies (Stamm, 1995, 2002) tend to support the existence of traumatoid states. There appears to be a direct relationship between the extent of exposure in professional roles to trauma patients and the presence of stress-evoked symptoms.

In a study of child protective service (CPS) workers, T. W. Meyers and T. A. Cornille (2002) documented a dose-response relationship between work stress and symptoms. They found that those who worked more than 40 hours per week had significantly higher rates of anger, irritability, jumpiness, exaggerated startle response, difficulty in concentrating, hypervigilance, nightmares and intrusive thoughts—as measured by the Impact of Events Scale: Revised for PTSD (Weiss, 1997, 2004; Wilson & Keane, 1997) and the Brief Symptom Inventory (Derogatis, 1975)—than those who worked less than 40 hours per week.

The researchers also measured the CPS worker's history of personal trauma and family of origin variables which assessed patterns of detachment and enmeshment based on Minuchin's model of family interaction. They found that 82% of the professional child care workers had a history of personal trauma prior to their professional employment. As expected, family of origin factors were associated with lifestyle patterns of adjustment and work-related stress. Professional CPS workers who grew up in detached families had withdrawn, isolated and "schizoid" lifestyles. In contrast, those raised in enmeshed families reported more symptoms of traumatoid states which included nightmares and intrusive memories related to their work responsibilities. Moreover, their findings included the data that 77% of the CPS workers reported that they had been assaulted or threatened on the job, and that those who witnessed a death had significantly higher levels of anxiety, hostility, paranoid ideation and overall severity of psychological symptoms. Somatic complaints (e.g., muscular pain and discomfort, cardio-vascular, gastrointestinal, breathing problems) were significantly more prevalent among the CPS workers who had experienced serious injury prior to working with child abuse victims. These results are consistent with the model of traumatoid states presented in Figure 8.1, where compassion fatigue is thought to develop out of work-related dysregulated affects.

In a study of extreme disaster, the 1995 terrorist bombing of the Oklahoma City Murrah Federal Building, David Wee and Diane Meyers (2002) examined stress-related reactions among 34 disaster mental health workers who were provided with questionnaires assessing compassion fatigue and symptoms of PTSD, using Calvin Frederick's Reaction Index and the SCL-90-R symptom checklist (Derogatis, 1975). The results indi-cated the presence of traumatoid states among the disaster workers at the site of the bombed building.

In examining the major findings, 64.7% of the workers reported PTSD symptoms on the Frederick Reaction Index, with 8.8% registering severe symptoms. Gender differences were found on the SCL-90-R symptom checklist. Males had higher scores on the global summary indices (GSI, PST, PSDI) than females, suggesting a greater degree of psychological dis-tress. Further, the length of exposure to disaster work was significantly cor-related with compassion fatigue and burnout, as measured by Figley's (1995) self-test. Of particular importance to our model (presented in chap-ter 8) is the finding of Wee and Meyers (2002) that "respondents who believed that someone they knew might die as a result of the bombing experienced significantly greater levels of empathy from people involved in the bombing experience" (p. 74). This result is consistent with Figure 8.3 which illustrates that empathic strains emanate from empathic identifica-tion, and are a precondition for traumatoid states, such as compassion fatigue and secondary traumatic stress reactions.

In an interesting study which has direct relevance to the data and conclusions to be presented in this chapter, Meldrum, King, and Spooner (2002) assessed secondary traumatic stress reactions in case managers who were working in 41 community mental health clinics in the five states and the Northern Territory of Australia. Meldrum and her colleagues used the secondary traumatic stress disorder scale (STSD) which converts the DSM-IV diagnostic criteria for PTSD into a nearly identical version to assess STS reactions. The sample of 300 respondents was subsequently classified into three groups based on their STS scores, using the same algorithm criteria for PTSD in the DSM-IV. The results showed that 17.7% met the full criteria for STSD; 18% were classified as subclinical; and 64.0% had no diagnosis, reflecting minimal or no symp-toms. In their conclusions, Meldrum et al. (2002) state that

> since there is a lack of normative data … comparison of the rates of STS we
> have recorded with those from other occupational groups is not possible … *it*

remains unclear as to the extent to which STS is best understood as a specific stress reaction and the extent to which it is better understood as a generalized stress condition. (p. 99, italics ours)

The researcher's conclusion fits well with Figure 8.3, in which it is proposed that occupational stress response syndromes (OSRS) derive from traumatoid conditions such as compassion fatigue, secondary traumatic stress and vicarious traumatization.

TRAUMATOID STATES: EMPIRICAL EVIDENCE FOR PROLONGED STRESS REACTIONS TO CLINICAL WORK WITH TRAUMA VICTIMS AND PTSD

The CTRS, described in chapter 9, was used to generate the information presented in Figures 10.1–10.12. To facilitate clarity in presentation, we will address the questions posed in chapters 8 and 9 by organizing the chapters into sections. Each section will present data from the CTRS which has relevance to the questions of *traumatoid states*: compassion fatigue, secondary traumatic stress reactions and vicarious traumatization. The larger issues of whether or not stress reactions associated with different forms of trauma work (e.g., psychotherapy, disaster response, first responders, crisis debriefers, ER physicians, etc.) are best considered as generalized stress reactions or OSRS will be discussed as well.

Symptoms of Post-traumatic Stress Disorder: Prime Diagnostic Criteria

I. PTSD A_2—Prime Criteria
The CTRS contained two items pertaining to the DSM-IV A_2 diagnostic criteria for PTSD (items 92 and 93). Figure 10.1 shows that 71.4% of the 345 respondents admitted to feeling threatened, unsafe or being fearful of their

CTRS Item	DSM-IV	Percentage Responding	
		Affirm (Yes)	Often/Always
92. I have felt threatened or unsafe due to the behavior of my trauma clients.	A_2	75.60	1.20
93. I have experienced fear of my trauma clients.	A_2	67.20	12.80
Mean =	2 items	71.40	7.00

Figure 10.1 PTSD A_2 diagnostic criteria: Fear, helplessness or horror. Copyright John P. Wilson, 2003.

clients. However, *only* 7.0% reported such reactions "often or always." The data suggests that while the majority of respondents experienced fears and threats with clients, it was not a frequent occurrence in their work.

II.   Reexperiencing Phenomena
As noted in chapter 9, Factor I of the CTRS was labeled "Intrusive Preoccupation with Trauma" and consisted of 25 items accounting for 22.5% of the variance measured. Figure 10.2 presents item endorsement for reexperience phenomena (i.e., DSM-IV "B" criteria). A total of 15 items are specific to the reexperiencing cluster of stress-related reactions to trauma work. On average, 63.65% of the respondents confirmed having such experiences, i.e., reliving stress-related trauma accounts of their clients. The highest reported reaction (90.5%) is for the B_4 criteria as assessed by the item, "I have felt overwhelmed by the trauma story of my client," which was experienced regularly by 59.9% of the participants. The least frequently endorsed item (32%) is for dissociative-like reactions (B_3) of feeling such as "I was living in a dream with surreal features." This response rarely occurred on a regular basis (1.5%), and may reflect the low occurrence of dissociative reactions among therapists. Overall, 15.41% of the study participants reported having any (B_1–B_5) reexperiencing reactions on a regular basis.

III.   Avoidance and Numbing Phenomena
Figure 10.3 indicates that 28 items specifically assessed avoidance and numbing criteria (DSM-IV "C" PTSD criteria). The results of the CTRS factor analysis found that Factor II—Avoidance and Detachment—contained 19 items which account for 6% of the variance. The results of the item endorsements further clarify the significance and meaning of this factor.

The results show that, on average, 68.96% of the respondents declared experiencing avoidance and numbing reactions, whereas only 15.10% reported having them "often or always." The item with the highest endorsement (91.0%) reflects the C_5 criteria (detachment): "I have a need to distance myself emotionally from my trauma client during sessions or when away from the office." The item with the lowest endorsement (8.4%) is, "I have purposely cancelled appointments to avoid dealing with my trauma clients." Further, of all the avoidance and numbing response categories, the C_3 (inability to recall) and C_5 (detachment) have the highest rates of endorsement (83.20% and 79.02%, respectively) and are the most likely to be experienced on a regular basis (22.70% and 21.52%, respectively). The item endorsements affirming the existence of the DSM-IV "C" criteria (C_1–C_7) ranged from 45.20% to 83.20%. The reported frequency of "often or always" was 1.50–22.70%, indicating considerable variability in the frequency of avoidance and numbing reactions to trauma work.

CTRS Item	DSM-IV	Percentage Responding	
		Affirm (Yes)	*Often/Always*
1. I have felt overwhelmed by my client's trauma story.	B_4	95.90	59.90
5. I have experienced difficulty controlling my feelings while listening to my client's trauma story.	B_4	85.10	28.80
63. After meeting with trauma clients I have difficulty getting the image of their trauma story out of my mind.	B_1	82.00	2.30
33. I have found myself haunted by my clients and their trauma stories.	B_1	74.40	34.10
81. In my professional work I experience vicarious traumatization.	B_{1-5}	72.80	3.80
86. The impact of the trauma work has caused me to feel "as if" I were living in a bad dream with surreal fears.	B_3	32.00	1.50
42. I have found myself reliving my client's flashbacks, dreams or traumatic memories.	B_{2-3}	38.40	7.00
64. I have felt "as if" I were reliving the experiences of my trauma clients.	B_1	38.60	6.70
41. I have been so emotionally charged from working with my trauma clients that it seemed "as if" I were the victim too.	B_3	49.00	1.80
48. I have experienced more stress and tension after meeting with my trauma clients.	B_5	84.90	8.40
50. I have experienced somatic reactions (e.g., bodily pain, throat conditions, muscle tension, etc.) during or after sessions.	B_5	59.20	4.40
53. I have experienced changes in my breathing patterns while listening to my client's trauma story.	B_5	65.80	7.00
54. I have experienced nausea while listening to my client's trauma stories.	B_5	34.20	13.00
76. After working with my trauma clients I have been preoccupied with thoughts and feelings about trauma and arms.	B_1	78.80	37.10
Mean =	14 items	63.65	15.41

Figure 10.2 Re-experiencing. Copyright John P. Wilson, 2003.

| CTRS Item | DSM-IV | Percentage Responding | |
		Affirm (Yes)	Often/Always
10. I have felt a need to distance myself emotionally from my trauma client during sessions or away from the office.	C_5	91.00	12.50
24. I have experienced emotional or empathic detachment while meeting with trauma clients.	C_5	89.50	44.20
29. I have questioned whether or not the reported trauma history was the real cause of my client's problems.	C_2	82.40	4.70
7. I have experienced the need to intellectualize the trauma story in order to avoid personal distress.	C_5	83.70	41.90
16. I have wanted to escape from my awareness of the disturbing content of my client's trauma story.	C_3	83.90	37.00
31. I have wished that prescribed medications would make my trauma client easier to work with.	C_2	81.30	22.30
80. I have found it difficult to disclose information to others about the horrific traumatic events I learn about.	C_1	79.30	23.20
81. I have felt that I cannot burden others with the traumatic events I have heard, so I keep them to myself and deal with them alone.	C_1	71.90	14.80
78. I have had difficulty remembering all that my trauma clients have told me.	C_3	82.50	8.40
25. I have had thoughts of referring my trauma clients to someone else for help	C_2	80.40	2.30
69. After meeting with my trauma clients I have experienced a sense that my life could be short or shortened.	C_7	64.10	8.80
67. I have felt a need to be alone after meeting with my trauma clients.	C_5	70.30	5.30
84. In my work with trauma clients I have experienced being "out of touch" with my own emotions or feelings.	C_6	74.50	4.10
6. While listening to my trauma clients I have felt a need to hide behind a professional role.	C_2	76.00	4.10

Figure 10.3 Persistent avoidance and numbing of general responsiveness. Copyright John P. Wilson, 2003.

CTRS Item	DSM-IV	Percentage Responding	
		Affirm (Yes)	Often/Always
13. I have found myself not wanting to believe my client's trauma story.	C_2	76.80	3.50
23. I have experienced the wish that my trauma client not show up for the scheduled appointments.	C_2	78.60	29.00
52. I have experienced myself "numbing out" while listening to my trauma clients.	C_6	69.20	31.10
26. There have been times when I have wished that I did not have to work with trauma clients.	C_2	67.70	29.00
51. I have found myself growing drowsy or sleepy while listening to my trauma clients.	C_5	67.30	26.40
90. I have been reluctant to speak honestly to colleagues/supervisors for fear of being viewed as a novice, inept or weak.	C_1	61.80	5.90
99. I believe that many clients malinger or fake their PTSD or trauma symptoms.	C_2	73.00	12.90
85. I have experienced a loss of sensuality and emotional sensitivity due to my immersion in trauma work.	C_6	62.10	4.40
62. I have found myself "steering" the conversation with trauma clients in the direction that makes me feel less distressed.	C_1	66.80	16.10
47. I have found myself using more alcohol and/or drugs after meeting with my trauma clients.	C_6	29.00	10.70
28. I have had thoughts of terminating therapy even though I knew there was more work to be done.	C_2	47.40	8.80
32. I have thoughts that my client's trauma story was not as bad as reported.	C_2	70.00	1.50
27. I have purposely cancelled appointments to avoid dealing with my trauma clients.	C_2	8.40	8.40
66. After meeting with my trauma clients I have experienced a loss of interest in activities I previously enjoyed.	C_4	45.20	1.50
Mean =	28 items	68.96	15.00

Figure 10.3 (continued)

CTRS Item	DSM-IV	Percentage Responding	
		Affirm (Yes)	Often/Always
49. Meetings with trauma clients have been stressful.	D_2	94.50	21.00
68. After being exposed to trauma stories I have experienced more concern for the safety of those I hold dear.	D_4	85.80	18.70
9. While listening to my trauma clients I found my attention lapsing and my thoughts drifting.	D_3	87.50	30.60
34. I have had strong emotional reactions to my trauma clients which lasted well beyond our meeting.	D_4	89.90	53.00
48. I have experienced more stress and tension after meeting with my trauma clients.	D_2	84.90	8.40
95. I have experienced an adrenaline rush or high while working with trauma clients.	D_4	70.10	7.00
59. After meeting with my trauma clients, I have found myself to be hypervigilant of what is happening around me.	D_4	68.60	31.10
46. I have experienced greater irritability and proneness to anger after meeting with my trauma clients.	D_2	62.90	2.60
45. After meeting with my trauma clients I have experienced an inability to fall asleep or stay asleep.	D_1	66.80	19.70
56. I have found myself reacting as my trauma client might (exaggerated startle response, on edge in crowds).	D_5	52.60	19.10
58. I have harbored resentment of my trauma clients for exposing me to the pain of their suffering.	D_2	23.50	0.60
55. I have found it difficult to concentrate on my client's trauma story as it was being told.	D_2	88.00	18.60
Mean =	12 items	72.91	19.20

Figure 10.4 Hyperarousal: Persistent symptoms of increased arousal. Copyright John P. Wilson, 2003.

IV. Hyperarousal: Persistent Symptoms of Increased Arousal not Present before Exposure

Figure 10.4 presents the results of the item endorsements that correspond to the DSM-IV "D" criteria, hyperarousal. Altogether, 12 items assessed these reactions during or after trauma work. Nearly all the respondents

(94.5%) affirmed that "meetings with my trauma client have been stressful." Similarly, 89.9% stated, "I have had strong emotional reactions to my trauma clients which lasted well beyond our meeting together." Likewise, 84.9% said that they had "experienced more stress and tension after meeting with my trauma clients."

On average, 72.91% of the participants affirmed experiencing hyperarousal reactions. Interestingly, from the perspective of empathic attunement, 87.5% of the respondents reported lapses of attention and drifting thoughts during sessions, and 30.6% stated that this occurred regularly (i.e., "often or always"). In other words, about one-third of therapists have difficulty in sustaining attention, and admit that their thoughts drift to other matters. On the other hand, only a few participants declared "harboring resentment" towards clients for being exposed to their pain and suffering (23.5% affirmed; 0.6% reported "often or always"). Nevertheless, 19.20% admitted to experiencing persistent reactions of increased arousal associated with their professional work.

V.   Summary of PTSD Criteria (A_2; B_{1-5}; C_{1-7}; D_{1-5}): Percentage Affirming ("Yes") any Symptoms and Those Reporting Reactions Frequently ("Often/Always")
Figure 10.5 offers a graphic summary of reported PTSD reactions to work with trauma clients, classified according to the DSM-IV diagnostic criteria for PTSD. The figure contains two columns showing the percentage of those with affirmative reactions ("yes"), and those who reported them as occurring frequently ("often/always"). Overall, 68.5% of the participants admitted to experiencing *any* PTSD-related reaction, and 16.57% reported experiencing them "often or always," a figure that closely matches Meldrum et al.'s (2002) figure of a 17.70% secondary traumatic stress rate among mental health supervisors in Australia.

Moreover, the range of reported PTSD-like reactions is remarkably consistent *within and among* diagnostic categories. For example, PTSD "B" (reexperiencing phenomena) range on a *regular basis* from 7.3–59.9%; PTSD "C" (avoidance and numbing), 1.50–22.70%; and PTSD "D," 10.24–30.60%. For respondents who admitted to experiencing any PTSD-like reactions, 68.50% confirm having had these reactions in the course of their work as therapists or mental health professionals. While PTSD reactions are not reported on a regular basis with great frequency, they do occur among a high percentage of therapists at some point during their professional work, both in and out of the office setting.

B—Symptoms of Vicarious Traumatization

I. Impact of Trauma Work on Professional Identity
Figure 10.6 presents the analysis of item endorsements reflecting the impact of trauma work on professional identity. The four items on the

A_1 – Professional Work with Trauma Patients and PTSD

A_2 – Fear, Helplessness and Horror (71.40% [affirm] 7.00% [often/always])

B - Traumatic Event (Client) is Persistently Reexperienced

	Affirm (Yes) %	Often/ Always %
B_1	63.93	34.56
B_2	38.60	7.00
B_3	40.50	1.65
B_4	90.50	59.09
B_5	63.38	7.30
Mean =	59.38	21.90

C – Persistent Avoidance of Stimuli Associated with the Trauma

	Affirm (Yes) %	Often/ Always %
C_1	69.95	15.00
C_2	62.45	11.50
C_3	83.20	22.70
C_4	45.20	1.50
C_5	79.02	21.52
C_6	58.70	12.57
C_7	64.10	8.08
Mean =	66.08	13.26

D – Persistent Symptoms of Increased Arousal

	Affirm (Yes) %	Often/ Always %
D_1	66.80	19.20
D_2	70.76	10.24
D_3	87.50	30.60
D_4	78.60	27.45
D_5	52.60	19.10
Mean =	71.25	21.31

Grand Mean (B, C, D) =	68.50	16.57

Figure 10.5 Summary of PTSD criteria endorsed on the CTRS. Copyright John P. Wilson, 2003.

CTRS that measured these attributes are listed in Figure 10.6. According to the data, 92.4% of the participants certified that "since working with trauma, I have felt that I am a different person now than I was before

	Percentage Responding	
CTRS Item	**Affirm (Yes)**	**Often/Always**
82. Since working with trauma I have felt that I am different now from how I was before I started to work with trauma clients.	92.40	53.80
37. I have felt like a liberator or savior in my helping role.	62.60	26.40
14. I have found myself wondering why I chose to work with trauma clients.	75.30	39.70
100. Due to the nature of my work with trauma clients I secretly wish I were doing something else.	48.00	3.20
Mean =	69.57	30.77

Figure 10.6 Impact of trauma work on professional identity. Copyright John P. Wilson, 2003.

I started to work with trauma clients." Similarly, 75.3% asserted that they questioned their motivation to do the work. Only a few respondents (3.2%) stated that "I secretly wish I were doing something else," and nearly 40% declared that they felt "like a liberator or savior in my helping role." Overall, 30.77% reported an identity-related impact, on a regular basis, associated with their professional work with trauma clients.

II. Impact of Trauma Work on Sense of Meaning, Worldview, Beliefs and Ideology
As noted by Pearlman and Saakvitne (1995), involvement in trauma work may lead to vicarious traumatization and alter self-capacities, including beliefs, values and systems of meaning. Figure 10.7 indicates that eight items on the CTRS are associated with this dimension of trauma work. All participants (99.9%) acknowledged that they "had been touched by their trauma client and their stories," and 83.2% reported that reaction "often or always." Understandably, 94.50% admitted to frustration that "society has not done more to prevent abuse and victimization." Perhaps for this reason, 89.2% stated that they "experienced a *deeper search for meaning* as to why victimization occurs." Almost the same percentage (89.5%) indicated that they found themselves reappraising "my own beliefs and values." Overall, 85.5% confirmed that the work they do had an effect on their sense of meaning, views of society, concept of victimization and the reason for engaging in professional work with trauma clients. Noteworthy, too, is the finding that 52.2% admitted to having "thoughts about avenging the wrongs committed against my trauma clients, although not on a regular basis" (4.4% = "often or always").

		Percentage Responding	
CTRS Item		**Affirm (Yes)**	**Often/Always**
89.	I am touched by my trauma clients and their stories.	99.20	83.20
70.	I have experienced frustration or anger that society has not done more to prevent abuse and victimization.	94.50	44.20
96.	I have experienced a heightened sense of meaning or reason for being when I do this work.	93.30	40.40
77.	Due to my work with trauma clients I have experienced a deeper search for meaning as to why victimization occurs.	89.20	33.70
60.	I have experienced disillusionment about the human condition due to work with trauma clients.	82.60	19.20
72.	After meeting with my trauma clients I have felt overwhelmed that there is evil, abuse and victimization in the world.	79.20	13.00
61.	Due to the impact of my trauma clients I have found myself re-appraising my own beliefs and values.	89.50	27.50
71.	I have found myself having thoughts about avenging the wrongs committed against my trauma clients.	52.20	4.40
Mean =		85.05	33.20

Figure 10.7 Impact of trauma work to sense of meaning, world view, beliefs and ideology. Copyright John P. Wilson, 2003.

C—Compassion Fatigue and Somatization

Somatic Reactions Manifest during Psychotherapy with Clients

Figure 10.8 lists the results of item endorsements on the CTRS for somatic reactions manifest during work with trauma clients. The most global of the somatic items (item 50) found that 59.20% recounted experiencing "somatic reactions (e.g., bodily pain, throat conditions, muscle tension, etc.) *during or after* sessions with clients," whereas only 4.4% reported these somatic reactions on a regular basis. Across the four CTRS somatic items, an average of 52.65% admitted to experiencing headaches, changes in breathing patterns or nausea while interacting with their clients.

Of all the somatic symptoms reported as "often or always," the most prevalent are headaches at 18.6%; this is followed by experiences of "nausea while listening to the trauma story of the client" (13.0%). Clearly, the

	Percentage Responding	
CTRS Item	**Affirm (Yes)**	**Often/Always**
44. During or after meeting with my trauma clients I have experienced *headaches*.	51.40	18.60
50. I have experienced *somatic reactions* (e.g., bodily pain, throat conditions, muscle tension, etc.) during or after sessions with my trauma clients.	59.20	4.40
53. I have experienced changes in my *breathing pattern* while listening to my patient's trauma story.	65.80	7.00
54. I have experienced *nausea* while listening to my trauma client's trauma story.	34.20	13.00
Mean =	52.65	10.00

Figure 10.8 Somatic reactions manifest during psychotherapy with trauma clients. Copyright John P. Wilson, 2003.

presence of headaches, muscle tension, throat conditions (e.g., "lump in throat"), changes in breathing patterns, and nausea are all symptoms of increased sympathetic nervous system activity which, if chronic or recurrent, could lead to states of fatigue, exhaustion, generalized discomfort and tension. In this regard, somatic reactions may be indicative of empathic identification with what clients report in their trauma narratives which then gets internalized by the therapist in the form of bodily manifestations.

D—Dysregulated Affects and Personal Reactions Associated with Trauma Work

We have suggested that empathic strain experienced during trauma work with clients is associated with states of dysregulated affects, as it is in chronic PTSD (Schore, 2003). Figure 10.9 lists the seven items on the CTRS that assess different forms of dysregulated affects, including fear, vulnerability, sadness, grief, mistrust and uncertainty. The results show that 78.90% of the respondents admitted to experiencing such reactions. Nearly all the participants reported experiencing uncertainty (94.5%) and "a deepened sense of sadness" (97.11%) connected with understanding the nature of what their clients endured in their personal traumas. Perhaps for this reason, 57.7% reported regularly experiencing states of "personal vulnerability while listening to the trauma stories of my clients." Finally, no matter what type of distressing affect was endorsed, 25.2% recounted experiencing these reactions "often or always" which seems to suggest their ubiquity in trauma work.

CTRS Item	Percentage Responding	
	Affirm (Yes)	Often/Always
2. I have experienced *uncertainty* as to my ability to work with my trauma clients.	94.50	7.60
3. I have experienced a sense of personal *vulnerability* while listening to my clients' trauma stories.	88.90	51.70
30. I have experienced *fear* that my trauma clients condition will have a *contagious* effect on me.	33.10	11.30
12. I have experienced *unwanted feelings and memories* from my past while listening to my trauma clients.	70.90	19.20
57. I have found myself *less trusting* of strangers since meeting with my trauma clients.	72.40	12.10
79. Because of my work with trauma clients I have felt a deepened *sense of sadness* at what some people are capable of doing.	97.10	48.20
83. I have experienced feelings of *grief, mourning and sadness* during or after meetings with my trauma clients.	95.40	26.40
Mean =	78.90	25.21

Figure 10.9 Dysregulated affect and personal emotional reactions associated with trauma work. Copyright John P. Wilson, 2003.

E—Professional Boundary Problems and Disclosure of Countertransference

The issues of boundary maintenance and disclosure of countertransference have been "red flagged" in discussions on the difficulties related to professional work with trauma clients, particularly in long term psychotherapy (Dalenberg, 2000; Pearlman & Saakvitne, 1995; Slatker, 1987; Wilson & Lindy, 1994). Four items on the CTRS assess professional boundaries with clients and disclosure of CTRs. Figure 10.10 shows the results of the data analysis, and indicates that 81.4% of the respondents reported difficulties in maintaining firm boundaries with their clients. A third (33.1%) of the participants indicated that this is a recurrent issue. In the light of these results, it is not surprising that 73.6% of the participants reported difficulty in "telling others a lot about the emotional impact of the work I do." Similarly, 61.8% admitted to a reluctance to speak honestly to colleagues or supervisors about their personal reactions for "fear of being viewed as a novice, inept or wrong."

Interestingly, however, whereas the professionals in our sample readily acknowledged experiencing "reluctance" to speak openly and honestly to colleagues and supervisors, only 5.9% indicated that they did this on a

CTRS Item	Percentage Responding	
	Affirm (Yes)	*Often/Always*
Professional Boundary Problems		
19. I have found it difficult to maintain firm bound-aries with my trauma clients due to the intensity of their need.	81.40	33.10
43. During meetings with my traumatized clients I have found myself struggling to maintain a professional role.	62.00	12.70
Mean =	71.70	22.90
Disclosure of Countertransference		
65. After meeting with my trauma clients, I experi-ence difficulty telling others a lot about the emo-tional impact of the work I do.	73.60	17.20
90. I have been reluctant to speak honestly to col-leagues/supervisors for fear of being viewed as a novice, inept or wrong.	61.80	5.90
Mean =	67.70	11.55

Figure 10.10 Professional boundaries and disclosure of countertransference. Copyright John P. Wilson, 2003.

regular basis. Therefore, while there are evident concerns about the maintenance of professional boundaries and the disclosure of personal reactions, the incidence of admitting to these concerns "often or always" is significantly lower, a fact that may reflect internal conflicts with regard to appropriate professional conduct in working with traumatized patients, whose personal histories of abuse often involve "boundary crossings" by perpetrators who demand secrecy about their behavior or, in case of default, inflict threats of reprisal (Herman, 1992, 1993). It is possible that these concerns about professional boundaries and disclosure of countertransference are a therapist's manifestation of being cast in a role by the clients and their enacting or reenacting the interpersonal dynamics for which they sought professional treatment.

F—Self-Disclosure of Personal Experiences in Trauma Work

If the respondents in our sample showed a reluctance to disclose to their supervisors personal difficulties associated with trauma work and the degree to which they are "emotionally impacted by the work," to whom do they self-disclose? Figure 10.11 summarizes the degrees of self-disclosure to different persons who include spouses, clergy, friends, colleagues, supervisors and others. Figure 10.11 indicates that the greatest

Persons Shared With...by Respondents	% of Respondents Who Share	Self-Disclosure		
		Small	Moderate	Great
Supervisor	46.70	11.30	14.80	20.60
Colleagues	91.90	12.20	40.00	39.70
Spouse/Significant Other	77.40	34.80	26.40	16.20
Minister (rabbi, etc.)	18.30	15.70	2.00	0.60
Family Member	34.50	23.80	9.00	1.70
Friend	53.40	26.40	20.60	6.40
Other	14.60	4.30	4.10	5.20
Share with No One	5.50	0	0	0

*Adapted from Wilson, Harel & Kahana (1989). In Wilson (1989), Trauma, Transformation and Healing: An Integrative Approach to Theory, Research and Post-Traumatic Therapy, New York: Brunner-Routledge.

Figure 10.11 Self-disclosure of personal experiences in trauma work. Copyright John P. Wilson, 2003.

degree of self-disclosure is to colleagues (91.9%) and spouses (77.4%). Further, self-disclosure to friends (53.4%) is greater than to supervisors (46.7%). Indeed, when analyzing the degrees of self-disclosure (small, moderate, great), we find that the results reveal nearly twice as much self-disclosure to colleagues (39.7%) as to supervisors (20.6%).

The findings from the CTRS are consistent with those concerning the management of professional role boundaries and disclosure of CTRs. The patterning of the results suggests the intriguing possibility that, while the therapists and trauma workers in our sample do self-disclose to their supervisors, they tend to disclose more to spouses, friends and professional colleagues, perhaps reflecting issues of trust, uncertainty, feelings of vulnerability and fears of appearing less than competent in their work. This raises an interesting question: Do trauma professionals have a unique tendency to suppress their inner states, doubts, fears and feelings of vulnerability? Dalenberg (2000) states that

> *suppression of affect* in the name of neutrality also could be a disguised version of posttraumatic stress disorder, the symptoms of which appear at clinically significant levels of those therapists who work with substantial numbers of trauma clients (Kassam-Adams, 1995). (p. 38, italics ours)

Since 78.90% of our sample confirmed experiencing affective states of sadness, fear, vulnerability, uncertainty and mistrust in the course of their work, are these emotions and affective experiences being suppressed in reports to supervisors, but shared with more intimate and trusted spouses, friends and peers? If such reticence exists, is it related in a causal or indirect way to the therapist's trauma history?

G—Incidence of Therapists with Personal Trauma History Treating Clients with Similar Trauma Histories

Analysis of demographic data revealed that 186 (54%) of the 345 participants in the CTRS study reported a history of personal trauma. Figure 10.12 presents the eight categories into which trauma workers with a personal history of trauma are classified, as gleaned from the demographic section of the CTRS (see demographic item 16, "Do you have a personal history of trauma?" with 24 choices which could be answered "yes" or "no"). The eight trauma categories are (1) emotional abuse in childhood or adulthood; (2) childhood sexual abuse; (3) medical trauma; (4) physical abuse in childhood or adulthood; (5) adult sexual assault; (6) spouse battering; (7) attempted suicide; and (8) war veteran shock. Figure 10.12 shows the correspondence between male and female clinicians, with a personal history of trauma, to the patient population they treat with the same history of trauma.

Overall, 88.50% of those with a personal history of trauma had been treating patients with a similar trauma history. For example, there is a 100% concordance for male veterans treating other male war veterans, whereas virtually no female clinicians treated war veterans. The lowest degree of concordance was that for medical trauma, where 74.0% had been treating patients with histories similar to their own.

While it is unclear whether or not these findings would be applicable to other samples of professionals working with trauma clients, the results strongly point to a motivational factor for choosing the trauma population that therapists elect to work with in a professional role. Clearly, this data is open to many interesting interpretations which include (1) therapists acquire empathic identification with clients by virtue of similar personal experience; (2) therapists have a conscious or unconscious desire to "work through" their own personal trauma by involvement with patients suffering similar traumas; (3) professionals have a perception of greater clinical efficacy in electing to work with patients whose trauma histories are readily understood and therefore with whom the professionals assume they can make a "better therapeutic connection"; (4) these therapists have a predisposition to Type II countertransference, overidentification, enmeshment and prosocial advocacy, posing both advantages and risks in their professional roles. In this regard, the third factor structure of the CTRS was labeled "Overinvolvement and Overidentification," the highest loading items of which are

- (.70) — I have experienced a protective attitude toward my client(s).
- (.64) — I have felt a strong urge to solve the problems of my trauma client(s).
- (.61) — I have thought of my client(s) as heroic for enduring the traumatic experience.

Personal Trauma History (Trauma Category)	Number of Female Clinicians with Personal Trauma History	Number of Female Clinicians Treating Same Trauma	Number of Male Clinicians with Personal Trauma History	Number of Male Clinicians Treating Same Trauma	Total Percentage of Clinicians Treating Clients with Same Trauma Type
Emotional Abuse (Child/Adult)	61	57	19	17	93
Sexual Abuse (Childhood)	48	42	10	10	90
Medical Trauma	37	28	10	7	74
Physical Abuse (Child/Adult)	25	23	10	8	89
Sexual Assault (Adult)	20	16	1	1	81
Battered Spouse	13	12	—	—	92
Attempted Suicide	8	7	1	1	89
Trauma of War Veterans	—	—	11	11	100
					Mean = 88.50

Figure 10.12 Incidence of therapists with personal trauma history treating clients with similar trauma histories. Copyright John P. Wilson, 2003.

- (.59) — I have experienced a need to protect, rescue or shelter my trauma client(s) from the abuses they have endured.
- (.53) — I have experienced concern for my trauma client(s) that extends beyond the work setting
- (.50) — I have done more for my trauma client(s) than is actually required by my profession.

It is evident that all of these items, loading on Factor III of the CTRS, reflect needs to protect and rescue the therapist's clients and solve their trauma-related problems, and also reflect the therapist's concerns that extend beyond the professional confines of the office space. Are professionals with a personal history of trauma more likely to manifest these behaviors with clients who "mirror" their own life experiences, and the psychological effects of which they dare produce to their self-capacities (Pearlman & Saakvitne, 1995)?

Discussion

What do the results of the study of professional members of ISTSS and ISSD tell us about stress responses to working with traumatized clients? Is there empirical support for the concepts of compassion fatigue, secondary traumatic stress, and vicarious traumatization? Is there any clinical or diagnostic significance in the concept of secondary traumatic stress disorder (STSD) as proposed by Figley (1995, 2002)? Are the reactions associated with difficulties in working with trauma patients more accurately embraced by the OSRS concept? Is the term *traumatoid states* a more inclusive and precise term, since it literally means "trauma-like" conditions which could characterize subclinical forms of PTSD, OSRS, and reactions of ordinary people to a broad range of stressful life events? In the most rudimentary sense, traumatoid states have the advantage of describing the outcome of exposure to stress-evoking situations of any type, not just professional role-related stress of psychotherapists, counselors, nurses, social workers, primary responders, ER doctors, crisis debriefers, disaster workers and others in helping occupations.

IS THE CONCEPT OF VICARIOUS PTSD OR SECONDARY TRAUMATIC STRESS DISORDERS VIABLE?

Is it clinically and scientifically meaningful to suggest that there are states of vicarious PTSD, secondary traumatic stress disorders (STSD) or states of vicarious traumatization? The answer appears to be "yes and no." The affirmative part of the answer rests in the strong evidence that those who work with trauma patients are clearly impacted by the work at multiple levels of psychological functioning. The therapists experience states of dysregulated affects, become preoccupied with their patients' trauma histories and powerful narratives of injury, abuse, and threat to physical and psychological existence. Exposure to trauma patients appears to have significant risk factors in terms of stress-related changes to self-capacities, beliefs, values, the meaning of life and understanding victimization. The risk factors of repeated, prolonged, or acute and intense exposure to trauma patients involves allostatic load and the need to understand how the human stress response system reacts to traumatic impacts to the organism (Wilson, Friedman, & Lindy, 2001).

A case can be made that medical and mental health professionals who have intensive and significant long-term involvement in trauma work will experience significant degrees of allostatic stress, as described by Bruce McEwen (1998) and discussed extensively by Wilson, Friedman, and Lindy (2001) in their book, *Treating Psychological Trauma and PTSD*. In PTSD, allostasis refers to the fact that traumatic events are at the extreme end of the stress continuum, and therefore the effects of exposure to life-threatening situations and so forth lead to a prolonged and chronic overactivation of the autonomic nervous system. The stress responses persist and the organism attempts to adjust. In doing so, it creates a new set point (baseline) for functioning and does not return to the pretrauma baseline functioning (i.e., homeostasis).

Moreover, the psychobiology of PTSD, as a form of prolonged stress response, seems to underlie the explicit rationale of the (A_1) PTSD, DSM-IV diagnostic criterion which states: "The person experienced, witnessed, or was confronted with an event or events that involved actual or threatened death or serious injury, or a threat to the physical integrity of self or others." This (A_1) PTSD diagnostic criterion clearly attempts to establish the definition of a traumatic stressor. In doing so, the criterion attempts to link different types of stressor exposure to behavioral response systems which include personal impacts; indirect exposure to horrific trauma (witnessing); and learning about or personally confronting the effects of a traumatic situation. These different types of exposure must involve death, threat of death, or injury to the self (i.e., victim) or others. Moreover, the second prime criterion (A_2) for diagnosing PTSD includes the emotional experience of "fear, helplessness or horror, or in children, disorganized or agitated forms of behavior."

IS PROFESSIONAL EXPOSURE TO TRAUMA CLIENTS A TRAUMATIC STRESSOR?

Allostasis is the psychobiological underpinning of PTSD symptoms. Once exposed to traumatic stressors, as characterized by the A_1 PTSD criterion, the stress response system "kicks into action" and manifests itself in an array of symptoms as adaptive (or maladaptive) stress responses. We must ask whether or not these same configurations of stress responses occur in psychotherapists, counselors, and others who are "one step removed" from the trauma experience, Is repeated exposure, over time, to trauma patients and their stories of abuse, victimization and survival *sufficient* to evoke allostatic stress response processes which operate in the exact psychobiological manner as direct traumatic exposure? Is professional exposure to trauma clients a traumatic stressor? Do cumulative effects summate, over time, to be functionally equivalent to a "Big Bang" traumatic event?

STRESSOR EXPOSURE ONE STEP REMOVED

To achieve a meaningful construct of STSD, four issues must be satisfied logically: (1) Does indirect (i.e., "second hand") or cumulative exposure lead to demonstrable stress-evoked symptoms in professionals exposed to client/patient trauma narratives, or their "in-person" presence in different clinical settings? (2) Do the configurations and profiles of psychobiologically based stress responses of therapists and others exposed secondarily to trauma match those of persons with firmly established PTSD diagnoses? (3) Do the psychobiologically based neurohormonal indices of PTSD (i.e., NE, 5-HT, DA, GABA, Cortisol, etc.) in secondary traumatic stress disorders match the configurations of trauma patients with positive diagnoses of PTSD? (4) Is there psychobiological evidence of morphological and functional changes in brain activity—similar to those of patients with a positive PTSD diagnosis—manifested by neuroimaging PET scans, MRIs and other measures of brain activity (Bremner, 2002)? (4a) Do psychometric assessments of PTSD in professional mental health workers match or resemble those of clients diagnosed with PTSD?

Currently, we have no studies that elucidate whether or not "secondary stress exposure" would, in fact, generate prolonged stress response syndromes similar to those of authentic PTSD. Moreover, Figley (2002) has defined STSD as "nearly identical to PTSD," and created diagnostic criteria that mimic those for PTSD. In order to establish some construct validity of STSD as "nearly identical" to PTSD would require satisfying the four aforementioned criteria. Equally important from a behavioral point of view is that, in the presence of STSD, the helpers would have to meet the A_2 PTSD diagnostic criteria of "fear, helplessness or horror." However, in neither of his publications (of 1995 and 2002) on compassion fatigue does Figley list any "nearly identical" A_2 diagnostic criteria for STSD. How then can there be a "nearly identical" pattern of STSD in PTSD without some means to establish comparability?

Moreover, the results of the CTRS revealed that, in terms of the A_2 PTSD criteria, *only* 7.0% reported experiencing reactions of "fear, helplessness or horror" on a regular basis (i.e., "often or always"). This means that 93% of our respondents *did not* consistently experience such stress responses. Nevertheless, 71.4% reported feeling threatened, unsafe or fearful in the course of their professional involvement with clients. But are such strong emotional reactions "front loaded" and occurrent more commonly at the beginning of treatment? Or are they more episodic in nature, depending on states of affect dysregulation in the clients associated with the latter's level of volatility?

The critical issue of satisfying logically defined criteria for the validation of the concept of STSD makes it difficult to determine if the other PTSD-like diagnostic criteria are part of a more generalized form of stress response to working with trauma clients. If it is not possible to establish the validity of the A_1 and A_2 stressor criteria for STSD, then what are we to make of the reports of reactions that are theoretically associated with the PTSD "B" (reexperience), "C" (avoidance) and "D" (hyperarousal) criteria? Are these genuine PTSD symptoms or *traumatoid reactions* similar to PTSD?

PATIENT AND THERAPIST REEXPERIENCING: ARE THEY THE SAME PHENOMENA?

In terms of the data reported on reexperiencing phenomena, several factors should be kept in perspective. First, 70% of the participants had over 10 years of professional experience in trauma work. Second, 70% of the sample were aged 46 or older. Third, 45.9% of the respondents had spent more than half of their professional time working with trauma clients, and nearly one-quarter work full time with such patients. Fourth, only 4.2% of the respondents reported having *more* than 10 hours of supervision per month, and 84.5% had *less* than 5 hours. These demographic data support the fact that the professionals under survey were older, well-experienced and received relatively little supervision. Keeping these facts in mind, what do such seasoned mental health professionals tell us about reexperiencing phenomena? Do they relive their patients' trauma stories and intense encounters in the office or clinical venue? The answer appears to be an unequivocal "yes."

In terms of reexperience phenomena, 63.65% admitted to experiencing such reactions and experiences. The strongest affect reported is "feeling overwhelmed," which is confirmed by 90.5% of the respondents and experienced on a regular basis by 59.9%. The second most frequently reported reaction concerns intrusive reliving experiences which were affirmed by 63.93%, and reported as regular by 34.56% of the participants. These data directly reflect the PTSD B_1 criteria of "persistent reexperience of the traumatic event." *In this case, what is persistently reexperienced are the patients' trauma stories, assessed by four items which are particularly noteworthy*:

- After meeting with trauma clients, I have difficulty getting the *image* of their trauma story out of my mind.
- I have found myself *haunted* by my trauma clients and their trauma history.
- I have felt "as if" I were *reliving* the experiences of my trauma clients.
- After working with my trauma clients I have been *preoccupied* with thoughts and feelings about trauma and abuse.

These items indicate the lingering presence of images that preoccupy and haunt the therapist; and, in some cases, they actually feel "as if" they are reliving what was told to them by the client.

It is interesting that the remaining reexperiencing symptoms (B_2, B_3 and B_5) were reported less than 8.0% of the time on a regular basis. So it would seem that, in terms of reexperiencing phenomena as a stress response, feelings of being overwhelmed and the persistence of the patients' accounts of their traumatic experiences are the most salient forms of reliving phenomena for the therapist. Moreover, 19.5% of the respondents stated that they regularly "experience concerns that extend beyond the office or work setting," and almost 95% recounted having such feelings at some point during their work with trauma clients. However, if nearly all the participants affirm having experiences concerned with their trauma clients that extend beyond the professional setting, how do they cope with these lingering reactions?

BLOCKING RECALL AND DETACHING: THERAPISTS' PRIMARY AVOIDANCE PATTERNS

Do psychotherapists manifest the same type of avoidance tendencies as do patients with PTSD? This question has important implications for understanding whether or not there is validity in the idea of compassion fatigue, or secondary traumatic stress reactions, or disorders as proposed by Figley (1995, 2002). In terms of PTSD, the criteria state that there is "persistent avoidance of stimuli associated with trauma and a general numbing of responsiveness *not present before the trauma.*" Symptoms include active forms of avoidance (C_1, C_2), amnesia or inability to recall aspects of the trauma experience (C_3), loss of interest in significant activities (C_4), forms of detachment from others (C_5), restricted ranges of affect (C_6), and attitudinal changes about the future (C_7). In a parallel way to analyzing PTSD avoidance symptoms, we can ask if there is evidence that therapists engage in similar avoidance behaviors associated with their work with trauma clients. The answer is both "yes" and "no."

The respondent data show that about the same percentage (68.96%) affirmed having avoidance reactions to their clients, at some point during the course of their work, as they did reexperiencing phenomena (63.65%). However, only 15.10% reported avoidance reaction of any type on a regular basis (i.e., "often or always"). More importantly, the two categories with the highest percentage of frequent avoidance behaviors fall into the C3 and C5 criteria: difficulty in remembering aspects of their clients' trauma stories (22.20%), and detachment (21.52%). These types of avoidance seem related to each other, considering that problems of recall concern memory, and detachment reactions reflect attempts to distance oneself from the client. It is also noteworthy that these two items load highly on CTRS Factor II, Avoidance and Detachment. The other types of PTSD-like avoidance behaviors (C_1, C_2, C_4, C_6 and C_7) are far less likely to occur on a regular basis, suggesting that the primary modalities of defensive avoidance are detachment, and "blocking out" memories of what the trauma clients report during clinical sessions. Does this mean that the content of the material being blocked out or forgotten is emotionally distressing and indicative of dysregulated affects?

The PTSD symptoms of hyperarousal ("D" criteria) are the most biological in nature, and reflect stress reactions to fear and threat which automatically trigger subcontrol emotional systems into operation (Friedman, 2000; LeDoux, 1996). The PTSD client's symptoms of increased arousal are reactive in nature and not present prior to the trauma on a regular basis. As part of a prolonged, allostatically changed pattern of organismic functioning, these symptoms of sleep disturbance, exaggerated startle response, hypervigilance, proneness to anger, irritability and problems of concentration are manifestations of disturbance in psychobiological equilibrium; a system that is running in an "overdrive" mode, "as if" the traumatic stressors were still present. However, since therapists are "one step removed" from the Big Bang of the client's traumatic experiences, do they manifest this same pattern of hyperarousal, even though they did not experience the original emotional state of fear and threat?

HYPERAROUSAL "ONE STEP" REMOVED FROM CLIENT TRAUMA

The results of the CTRS suggest that therapists regularly have strong emotional reactions to their clients which include problems in concentration (30.6%), sleep disturbances (19.20%) and hypervigilance (27.75%). The CTRS items which assessed reactions indicate that indices of increased arousal extend beyond the office setting. For example, "*after* meeting with my trauma clients, I have found myself to be *hypervigilant* of what is happening around me" (31.1%), and "I have had strong emotional reactions to my trauma clients that *lasted well beyond* our meeting together" (53.0%). Further, 94.5% of the participants asserted that "meetings with trauma clients have been stressful," and 21.0% stated that this occurs "often or always." Taken as a set of findings, there appears to be ample evidence that work with trauma clients is associated with increased arousal, dysregulated affect, and impacts to sleep patterns, cognitive processes (attention, hypervigilance) and reactions to unexpected stimuli (exaggerated startle response).

Are the magnitude and intensity of these symptoms of hyperarousal in therapists the same as they are in patients with a positive PTSD diagnosis? Would therapists generate identical types of "biological markers" of hyperarousal as do PTSD patients in tests, comparing neurohormonal evidence of PTSD? Would therapists show the same pattern of changes in cortisol, norepinephrine, serotonin (5-HT) as has been documented in studies of PTSD patients (Bremner, 2002; Friedman, 2000)? Is hyperarousal one step removed from the client's trauma the same type of hyperarousal? Is it only a matter of degree in hyperarousal that differentiates clients and therapists at the psychological response level?

TRAUMA WORK AND VICARIOUS TRAUMATIZATION: IS THERE A LASTING IMPACT TO SELF-CAPACITIES?

Vicarious traumatization is a concept developed by Laurie Anne Pearlman and Karen W. Saakvitne in their book, *Trauma and the Therapist* (1995). Vicarious traumatization, like secondary traumatic stress, implies that the therapist gets traumatized vicariously through exposure to trauma patients. Pearlman and Saakvitne's work stemmed primarily from work with incest survivors, children subjected to many forms of exploitation, abuse, developmental injuries, and loss of normalcy in healthy attachments and interpersonal boundaries pertaining to love, affection and sexuality. Pearlman and Saakvitne have documented the difficulties in working with adult survivors of childhood incest and noted that, beyond the technical difficulties in psychotherapy, the intense work with this population of trauma survivors has a strong potential to generate emotional impacts on the therapist. They coined the term *vicarious traumatization* to characterize the different ways in which therapists can become emotionally distressed. They suggest that therapist self-capacities are changed through the *cumulative effects* of intense trauma work with incest survivors, and that these changes may be *permanent*; that doing the work of post-traumatic therapy, over a significant period of time, molds impressions into the fabric of the therapist's inner self, much as children mold impressions into blocks of clay. To quote,

> When these [self-capacities] are impaired by vicarious traumatization, the therapist can be overwhelmed with *dysphoric feelings, self-criticism,* and *anxiety.* He may find it more difficult to be alone without feeling *anxious, depressed* or lonely; to tolerate and integrate strong feelings; to hold on to images of loving others; to enjoy activities or people previously valued. *The therapist may feel sorrow, grief, anger or rage.* His tears may be very close to the surface much of the time … the traumatized therapist may find it more difficult to calm and soothe himself and may turn to external sources of comfort, relief, or numbing, such as alcohol consumption, overeating, overspending, overwork, and television. (p. 288, italics ours)

What do the results of the CTRS tell us about vicarious traumatization? Do they support the concept of vicarious traumatization, and changes in therapist self-capacities as attributed to post-traumatic therapy? The answer is "yes, quite a bit."

In terms of the impact of trauma work on a sense of professional identity, 69.57% affirmed that it had influenced some aspect of their sense of themselves professionally, and had affected their sense of meaning, beliefs, values and worldview (85.5%). For example, an impressive 92.4% of the participants asserted that "since working with trauma, I have felt that I am different now from how I was before I started to work with my trauma clients." Nearly two-thirds (62.60%) testified that they "have felt like a liberator or savior in my helping role." However, doing post-traumatic therapy had led to self-doubt and uncertainty. Three-fourths (75.30%) of the participants confirmed that they found themselves "wondering why I chose to work with trauma clients," and about one-half (48.0%) affirmed that they have "secretly wished I were doing something else." This self-questioning is very likely related to the fact that all the participants attested that they have been "touched by my trauma clients and their stories."

The consequences of "being touched" by their clients' trauma stories is important, because it appears to have contributed to changes in worldview, search for meaning in life and a disposition towards prosocial advocacy, an observation made by Wilson and Lindy (1994). Evidence of changes in these aspects of therapist self-capacities may be seen in the following item endorsements:

- Due to the impact of my trauma work with clients, I have found myself *reappraising* my own beliefs and values (89.5%).
- I have experienced a heightened *sense of meaning* or reason for being when I do this work (93.3%).
- I have experienced *disillusionment* with the human condition due to work with my trauma clients (82.6%).
- Due to my work with trauma clients, I have experienced a deeper *search for meaning* as to why victimization occurs (89.2%).
- I have experienced *frustration or anger* that society has not done more to prevent abuses and victimization (94.5%).

These data suggest that, through the process of work with trauma clients, the professionals not only feel differently about themselves from the way they did before post-traumatic therapy—thus undergoing an identity change—but they are also forced, by the intensity and nature of the work, to feel disillusioned and to reappraise their own beliefs and values. However, the process of being transformed by the work in a specific way leads to a dual-edged sword of emotional experience. On the one edge of the trauma-sharpened sword is a heightened sense of meaning and purpose for being, as a person. As noted by Pearlman and Saakvitne (1995), the work is intrinsically fulfilling, and leads to satisfaction at doing something good, helpful and meaningful for the lives of patients severely injured by violations of their human integrity through incest traumatization. On the other edge of the sword, it is the therapist's personal struggle to understand how such victimization occurs. For example, in terms of incest, therapists ponder how parents can treat their children as objects of exploitative use for selfish satisfaction? How could parents violate the seraphic sanctity of childhood by sexual abuse, or ensnare their children into twisted and demonic relationships in the name of love? How could parents repeatedly engage the innocence of their children only to destroy it for a lifetime? The trauma stories of such patients bring to life and to full animation the horrific, incredible reality of these insidious forms of childhood abuse.

The same saga of struggle with evil is applicable to therapists who work with victims of torture, war, disaster, spousal battering and other types of trauma. For example, when we present the case histories of Teresa, the torture victim, the Bosnian widow of ethnic cleansing, or the Vietnam veteran picking brains out of his combat boots, it impacts anyone who hears these chronicles, often in distressing ways, even in the safety and comfort of a classroom. And yet these narratives are removed "three steps" from the original situation in which a therapist and a patient sit together in a room, sharing the preserved emotional reality of the trauma. If such accounts are distressing to those who hear and experience them "second, third or fourth hand," at a safe distance from the victim, is it not to be expected that the responsible professional engaged in post-traumatic therapy would experience dysregulated affective reactions and somatic symptoms as part of the work?

DYSREGULATED AFFECTS AND SOMATIC REACTIONS ASSOCIATED WITH TRAUMA WORK

If the concepts of secondary traumatic stress and vicarious traumatization have validity, then dysregulated affects and somatic reactions are "mirrored" stress responses in the therapist. In PTSD, dysregulated affective states are an integral part of the right-brain generated emotional patterns. Allan N. Schore's (2003) exhaustive literature review and synthesis states,

> Indeed, there is now evidence to show that early relational trauma is partic-
> ularly expressed in right hemisphere deficits. Very recent studies reveal that
> maltreated diagnosed with PTSD manifest right lateralized metabolic limit
> abnormalities ... and that right brain impairments associated with severe
> anxiety disorders are expressed in childhood. Adults severely abused in child-
> hood and diagnosed with PTSD show reduced right hemisphere activities
> during a working memory task. Neurological studies confirm that dysfunc-
> tion of the right frontal lobe is involved in PTSD symptomatology. (p. 153,
> references cited in original paragraph deleted for continuity in reading)

Schore's research provides solid scientific evidence of the critical activity of the right brain hemisphere in PTSD, anxiety disorders and manifestations of fear and anxiety states associated with dysregulation in the limbic system and especially the amygdala.

The relevance of these findings to therapists working with trauma clients is the possibility that, through intense exposure to trauma clients with diagnoses of PTSD, dissociative disorders, anxiety disorders and self-pathologies (i.e., borderline), the therapists themselves begin to experience dysregulated affects. This is what we mean by the phrase "mirrored stress responses."

The results of the CTRS provides evidence of the presence of dysregulated affects and somatic reactions in therapists. Among these affective states, sadness, grief, mourning and vulnerability are predominant, with 92.67% confirming these reactions to their work with trauma clients. Additionally, one-third affirmed experiencing fear that their trauma clients' condition (e.g., PTSD, dissociative disorders, etc.) would have a *contagious* effect on them. When analyzing the persistence of emotional reactions that occur "often or always," feelings of vulnerability (51.7%) and a sense of sadness (48.20%), associated with the awareness of malevolence in perpetrators, stand out among the others.

It is possible to speculate that the dysregulated affects experienced by trauma therapists are related to somatic reactions. If persistent exposure to trauma clients with chronic stress disorders (e.g., PTSD) leads to periods of intense affect dysregulation, we expect that it will be internalized in somatic ways. The results of the CTRS show that, on average, 52.65% of the participants testified to experiencing somatic reactions (e.g., headaches, nausea, changes in breathing patterns) and 10.0% reported that they experienced them on a regular basis. However, among those respondents reporting frequent somatic reactions, the most prevalent symptom was headaches (18.6%).

Why headaches? Are headaches a form of "affect signal" to the therapist about the patient's internal working model? Are headaches a signal of empathic strain and loss of attunement, or the product of hyperarousal, muscle tension and an unconscious defense against feeling overwhelmed? Could headaches be a somatic form of defense which distracts attention from outwards (i.e., from the patient) to inwards (to the therapist's internal state)? Might headaches be a somatic signal that the therapist has reached the maximum level of information in processing the client's interactional dynamic? Or, finally, are headaches an affect signal of threats to therapist self-capacities? To once again quote Allan N. Schore's book *Affect Regulation and the Repair of the Self* (2003), in terms of principles of psychotherapeutic treatment,

> It is possible to have a conception of defense mechanisms as *non-conscious strategies of emotional regulation for avoiding, minimizing, or converting affects that are too difficult to tolerate*, with an emphasis on dissociation and projective

identification; these right brain *defenses present the entrance into "dreaded states"* changed with intense affects that can potentially traumatically disorganize the *self-system*. (p. 280, italics ours)

This quotation from Schore refers, of course, to the development of PTSD and dysregulated pathologies associated with trauma. However, does it apply equally well to some trauma therapists? Do trauma workers in general, and post-traumatic therapists in particular, run the risk of experiencing distressing and overwhelming dysregulated affects (i.e., fear, vulnerability, uncertainty, sadness, grief) which lead them to use defenses as "non-conscious strategies" of emotional regulation for avoiding, minimizing or converting affects that are too difficult to tolerate? Are such defensive and adaptive tendencies part of the psychological domain and territory of vicarious traumatization?

TRAUMA THERAPIST AND TRAUMA CLIENTS: WHO CHOOSES WHOM?

In our sample of 354 respondents from the membership rosters of ISTSS and ISSD, 54% reported a personal history of trauma, primarily childhood abuse. As Figure 10.12 shows, there are also other professional clinicians who were war veterans, battered spouses and survivors of medical trauma which is associated with illness or surgical procedures. The results of the survey reveal that 88.50% of the therapists, on average, were treating patients who had suffered the same types of abuse and trauma as the therapists had endured. The strength of this concordance of trauma history and background facts between therapists and clients is interesting, and raises several questions pertaining to our other findings on vicarious traumatization, affect dysregulation and PTSD-like symptoms reported by the participants.

First, do therapists consciously choose to work with patients whose history is similar to their own? If so, what effects do the therapists' background of trauma have on their dispositional propensities during the course of psychotherapy? For example, do they have their own histories of trauma and abuse rekindled by exposure to their clients' trauma narratives? Are they prone to Type II overidentification as a countertransference modality? Are they "at risk" of professional role boundary violations? Are they more secretive and nondisclosing of their stress-related reactions to patients, because of their own personal history of trauma and abuse?

Second, do therapists with a history of trauma possess more empathic capacity, resonance and stamina than therapists without a trauma history? Are "survivor" therapists analogous to members of alcoholics anonymous who share common problems in an arena of acceptance and commitment to recovery?

Third, are therapists with a personal history of trauma more predisposed to affect dysregulation and somatic reactions? Given the therapists' personal history of trauma, do they have a preexisting state of right-brain governed deficiencies in emotional regulation? Do they have a lowered threshold for "triggers" which would activate powerful dysregulated affects? Are they more vulnerable to exposure to intense trauma clients whose fantasies contain parallels to the therapists'own? Alternatively, are they more resilient, flexible and able to conceptualize therapeutic objectives with greater clarity and focus because of their own trauma experiences and empathic identification with the client? Clearly, these and related questions require study, and have the potential to provide insight into the complex nature of interpersonal dynamics in the course of psychotherapy.

PROFESSIONAL ROLE BOUNDARIES AND DISCLOSURE OF COUNTERTRANS-FERENCE

The issues surrounding professional role boundaries and the disclosure of countertransference have been the subject of research and clinical debate (Dalenberg, 2000; Hedges, 1992; Maroda, 1991; Slatker, 1987; Wolstein, 1988) which are not reviewed here. However, several key points from research conducted with therapists working with trauma and PTSD merit highlighting.

The four items on the CTRS that measured reports of concerns with professional boundaries and difficulties in self-disclosure of countertransference show nearly identical results. On average, 71.7% of the respondents affirmed difficulties in maintaining professional role boundaries with their clients, and one-third (33.1%) admitted to experiencing such difficulties regularly. Moreover, nearly one-quarter (22.90%) stated that they experienced difficulties with boundaries on a regular basis. Second, in terms of self-disclosure, 17.2% recounted "difficulty telling others a lot about the emotional impact of the work I do." A smaller percentage, 5.9%, admitted that they were reluctant to speak to colleagues or supervisors "for fear of being viewed as a novice, inept or wrong."

Taken as a set of findings, the item endorsements for boundary issues and self-disclosure appear to be interrelated. If it is difficult, at some point in time during treatment, to maintain "firm boundaries with trauma clients due to the intensity of their needs," then it might be equally difficult to disclose the feelings and reactions to supervisors or colleagues. As Figure 10.11 indicates, therapists report disclosing more of their professional concerns, and personal reactions to their work, to spouses (77.4%) and colleagues (91.4%) than to their designated supervisor (46.7%). In fact, the data show that they are *twice* as likely to self-disclose to colleagues as they are to supervisors, especially at higher levels of disclosure.

The advantages and disadvantages of disclosing countertransference has long been debated in psychoanalytic literature (see Maroda, 1991, and Slatker, 1987, for discussions). In the area of post-traumatic therapy, the issue remains clouded, not well understood or unresolved by empirical data. Dalenberg (2000) has rightly noted the dangers associated with the suppression of countertransference to the therapist's emotional well-being as well as to the emotional fabric of therapy itself:

> uninvolved therapists tend to report boredom and burn-out ... this style [cf. detachment] can put therapists at risk for dissociative symptoms, in which the feelings that are suppressed during daily clinical hours are acted out in extra therapeutic settings. (p. 38)

Pearlman and Saakvitne (1995) echo this theme in their discussion of therapist disclosure and the therapeutic frame in working with trauma patients:

> Thoughtful countertransference disclosure is a useful tool in psychotherapy with adult survivors of childhood sexual abuse. Because these clients come to any new relationship with assumptions based upon their experiences in early exploitative, abusive, and non-nurturing relationships, the use of the new therapeutic relationship to undo old patterns and create new ways of relating is a critical component of psychotherapy. (p. 158)

Future research needs controlled studies that carefully evaluate the conditions under which countertransference disclosures are beneficial to ongoing clinical treatments of trauma clients. Dalenberg's (2000) questionnaire study represents one approach to these critical issues in work with patients suffering from trauma and PTSD. Reflecting on our data in the light of the paucity of research studies in the area of post-traumatic therapy, we ask: Is the absence of empirical data on professional role boundaries and their relationship to countertransference self-disclosure a form of avoidance behavior itself and reflective of a generalized stress syndrome in therapists?

TRAUMATOID STATES: A GENERALIZED OCCUPATIONAL STRESS RESPONSE SYNDROME?

We believe that empathy is the key to understanding the phenomena described as compassion fatigue, secondary traumatic stress and vicarious traumatization. Empathic attunement and empathic identification with the trauma client are indigenous to trauma work and post-traumatic therapy. As discussed in chapter 5, empathic strains challenge the therapists' capacity to stay empathically attuned and to maintain their own psychological equilibrium during the course of treatment. This is the dilemma of the "balance beam" of empathy. However, this is not always possible. Our research has shown that therapists experience dysregulated affective states associated with exposure to the trauma narratives of their patients. They freely report PTSD-like symptoms associated with three factors: (1) the patient's accounts of trauma; (2) the patient as a person who presents—in the sanctity of the therapist's office—pain, suffering, confusion, discouragement, loss of trust and hope, feelings of being "damaged goods" and, in many cases, a diminished sense of self-worth and human dignity; (3) reactions to the historical and situational context in which abuse and traumatization occurred (e.g., warfare, family, political oppression, terrorist attack, genocide, marriage, natural disaster, in the line of duty, etc.). As a result of these three factors and the multitude of inherent stressors, the therapist experiences empathic strains which may then be manifest in the form of compassion fatigue, secondary traumatic stress reactions (i.e., PTSD-like reactions) and vicarious traumatization.

We believe that empathic identification and empathic strains, reflective of affect dysregulation in the therapist, may be connected with specific behavioral manifestations which include physical and mental fatigue (compassion fatigue); the acquisition of traumatoid states (i.e., PTSD-like reactions or secondary stress reactions); and transformations in self-capacities (vicarious traumatization). These types of reactions are interrelated forms of OSRS which have a broad range of impacts on personal and professional functioning. Figure 8.1 illustrates these professional outcomes: (1) the existence of OSRS; (2) countertransference processes; (3) somatization, fatigue, exhaustion; (4) impacts to self-capacities, including identity, beliefs, values, ideology, worldview; (5) the quality of interpersonal and affiliative patterns; (6) a search for meaning about trauma-related issues of morality, justice, fairness, authority, power, religion, salvation/redemption, atonement; and (7) spirituality and understanding the numinous experience.

The CTRS which was conducted with experienced mental health professionals who work with traumatized clients suffering from PTSD, dissociative disorders and self-pathologies has produced research evidence that aids the understanding of the important differences between the theoretical constructs of compassion fatigue, secondary traumatic stress (i.e., PTSD-like states) and vicarious traumatization. We are grouping these together under the rubric of OSRS.

We will attempt to provide a panoramic overview of the central issues in professional work with trauma clients. This panoramic overview is a broad image of the psychic landscape of human trauma. It is like viewing images of the azure-blue and white parts of the earth from a space shuttle: as the earth gets closer, the previously unclear geographic shadings and boundaries of oceans, land masses, deserts and mountain ranges gradually come into view. And with the continuing approach towards the planet, a telescopic-like resolution of the details of the earth may be seen in its entirety, as the earth rotates on its axis, spinning in space and governed by the forces of gravity. In a similar manner, we can observe the processes of working with traumatized clients from afar and gradually focus, in greater resolution, on the images of the psychic landscape of trauma-related medical and psychological states. And, like an astronaut exploring the surface of the moon in a new gravitational environment, the professional working with traumatized clients gets exposed to the textures and terrain of a vast and often unknown environment of psychic traumatization.

Traumatoid states, as OSRS, include the domain of emotional, psychological and interpersonal processes in work with victims of trauma. "Traumatoid" connotes "trauma-like" reactions, feelings, perceptions, thought processes, physiological reactions, interpersonal processes and self-capacities. Traumatoid states include what has been referred to as compassion fatigue, secondary stress reactions and disorders, and vicarious traumatization. Such states are unique as stress response syndromes, because they contain many specific features that develop directly from professional work with trauma clients, especially in terms of restorative psychotherapy efforts.

Traumatoid states are multidimensional in nature and exist on a continuum of severity. The following dimensions of traumatoid states are presented in Figure 10.13:

- Dysregulated affective states which include anxiety, fear, sadness, grief, anger, rage, uncertainty and persistent feelings of vulnerability.
- Empathic identification with trauma victims.
- Empathic strain and distress in work to assist traumatized clients.
- Somatic symptoms which include fatigue, headache, muscle tension, agitation, irritability, trembling, restlessness, sleep disturbances, problems of concentration and attention, dizziness, nausea, tachycardia, changes in breathing patterns, etc.
- Altered self-capacities in terms of identity, self-care, sense of meaning, beliefs, attitudes, values, ideology and worldview.
- Personal reactions to trauma victims, during professional work, which may be positive or negative in nature. In psychotherapy, these are traditionally identified as countertransference processes.
- Difficulties in describing and disclosing the impact of the work to others.
- Altered stress tolerance thresholds and coping patterns.
- Allostasis and allostatic load phenomena.
- Altered conceptions of spirituality, the meaning of life-death, the soul and the numinous experience.

**TRAUMATOID STATES ARE MULTIDIMENSIONAL
STRESS RESPONSE SYNDROMES**

1. Dysregulated affective states which include anxiety, fear, sadness, grief, anger, rage, uncertainty and persistent feelings of vulnerability.
2. Empathic identification with trauma victims.
3. Empathic strains and distress in work in assisting traumatized clients.
4. Somatic symptoms which include fatigue, headaches, muscle tension, agitation, irritability, trembling, restlessness, sleep disturbance, problems of concentration and attention, dizziness, nausea, tachycardia, and changes in breathing patterns.
5. Altered self-capacities associated with personal identity, self-care, sense of meaning, beliefs, attitudes, values, ideologies and worldview.
6. Personal reactions to trauma victims during treatment which may be positive or negative in nature. In psychotherapy these reactions are identified as countertransference processes.
7. Difficulties in describing and disclosing the impact of the work to others.
8. Altered stress tolerance thresholds and coping patterns.
9. Allostasis and allostatic manifestations of stress response.
10. Altered conceptions of spirituality, life and death, the soul and the numinous experience.

Figure 10.13 The dimensions of traumatoid states as occupationally related stress response syndromes. Copyright John P. Wilson, 2003.

DEFINITION AND DIAGNOSTIC CRITERIA OF TRAUMATOID STATES

Traumatoid states are resultant psychological conditions that develop by active professional involvement with trauma clients, or by significant exposure to traumatized persons. Traumatoid states are syndromes of interrelated stress response processes, including a range of reactions, symptoms and behavioral tendencies. As OSRS, traumatoid states are related to empathic identifications with the physical and psychological injuries of traumatized persons. Empathic identification with the status of the trauma victim is frequently associated with empathic distress, and then experienced as different forms of affect dysregulation which include fear, anxiety, anger, rage, sadness, grief, numbing and persistent feelings of vulnerability. Traumatoid states may be transient, acute or chronic in nature and vary in severity. They may be episodic in nature and reactivated by contact with persons, situations or stimuli associated with the precipitating experiences of exposure to traumatized patients. In addition, repeated or prolonged exposure to traumatized persons may result in allostatic manifestations of stress response and an altered threshold of coping, difficulty in tolerating other stressors, and problems with self-monitoring internal states of arousal, affects and thought processes.

Traumatoid states may also be manifest in somatic reactions (e.g., fatigue, muscle strain, headaches, etc.).

The development of traumatoid states is also related to therapists' inability or unwillingness to disclose what they are feeling or experiencing as a consequence of exposure to traumatized others. Exposure to certain forms of traumatization (e.g., torture, childhood abuse) is linked with impacts to therapist self-capacities, belief systems, values and worldview, including religious and spiritual orientation. Traumatoid states may cause clinically significant impairment of social relations, occupational or other areas of functioning. Some occupations are more likely than others to pro-mote traumatoid states, for example, long term psychotherapy with patients suffering from post-traumatic stress disorders, self-pathologies (e.g., borderline personality disorders) and dissociative disorders; occupa-tions involving emergency and first-responders, and disaster workers in catastrophic situations leading to death, dying, chaos and destruction.

The definition and classification of traumatoid is presented in Figure 10.14.

THE CONCEPTUAL PARSIMONY OF TRAUMATOID STATES

Is there an advantage in utilizing the concept of traumatoid states instead of compassion fatigue (CF), secondary traumatization (STS) and vicarious traumatization (VT)? If so, what are the advantages of using the construct of traumatoid states in research, clinical training and education?

First, the construct of traumatoid states is parsimonious and encom-passes all of the phenomena previously studied under the rubrics of CF, STSD and VT. Second, unlike Figley's definition of STS as "nearly identi-cal" to PTSD, the concept of traumatoid states eschews the seemingly log-ical necessity of placing professional clinical work or duty-related stressors into a PTSD framework. As we noted earlier, professionals who work with trauma clients *do not* directly experience either the A_1 or the A_2 PTSD prime diagnostic criteria.

To review, *only* 7% of the respondents reported feelings of fear, threat or being unsafe on a regular basis—the emotional reactions typically associated with Big Bang trauma experiences. Further, none of the profes-sionals in our sample has experienced, through exposure to their clients, an event or ordeal that would qualify or resemble the stressor dimensions normally connected with "first hand" traumatic experience, that is, the A_1 PTSD diagnostic criteria. Second- or third-hand exposure is *not* a Big Bang stressor event. However, as noted in the discussion on proposed diagnos-tic criteria for traumatoid states, some professional workers (e.g., first responders, EMT, disaster rescue professionals, ER personnel) may have *direct exposure* to traumatic events per se and therefore be at risk of both

A The person has been exposed to a traumatized individual who has experienced physical and psychological injuries as a result of professional work or by significant personal experience on a regular basis with such person(s).

B Following significant exposure to a traumatized persons, people develop symptoms of dysregulated affect, somatic reactions, hyperarousal, and tendencies to reexperience or avoid traumatized persons' reports of their physical or psychological injuries which were *not present* before such exposure.

C As a result of exposure to traumatized persons, people undergo alterations in psychological functioning which are manifest in self-capacities, stress tolerance, worldviews, belief systems, values, ideologies, religious and spiritual orientation which were *not present* before such exposure.

D Traumatoid states may be transient, acute or chronic in nature and characterized by recurrent episodes which may vary in severity and duration.

E Traumatoid states may cause clinically significant impairment or distress in social, occupational or other areas of functioning.

Figure 10.14 Diagnostic criteria for traumatoid states and occupationally related stress response syndromes. Copyright John P. Wilson, 2003.

PTSD and traumatoid states. Similarly, the prolonged cumulative effects of trauma work may "summate" and begin to function psychologically as a Big Bang trauma event.

At present, there is no scientific data to support the idea that STS is "nearly identical" to PTSD in its etiology, psychobiology, sequela, and functioning within the brain. However, this does not rule out the possibility that *cumulative traumatic exposure* to trauma clients who suffer physical and psychological injuries and/or disorders may not have effects *similar* to PTSD. Clearly, this is an empirical issue. For example, do therapists who work full time with trauma clients show the same types of changes in neurohormonal functioning as PTSD-positive patients? Do these therapists manifest patterns of brain changes in morphology and functioning identical to those evidenced in neuroimaging studies of PTSD? Do therapists dealing with trauma patients register psychometric data consistent with profiles of PTSD on objective and projective measures (see Wilson & Keane, 2004)? Without substantive empirical data to confirm the psychobiological and psychometric similarities between PTSD-positive clinical cases and cases of STSD, the concept of such reactive patterns being "nearly identical" to PTSD is without scientific merit.

DO WE NEED A NEW DSM-V DIAGNOSTIC CATEGORY FOR TRAUMATOID STATES?

The proposed definitional criteria for traumatoid states as OSRS do not require that they meet "nearly identical" A_1 or A_2 prime criteria for PTSD or any other symptoms of the anxiety disorder. Instead, the former criteria require only that the "person has been exposed to a traumatized individual who has suffered physical or psychological injury as a result of professional work or by significant personal exposure on a regular basis to such persons." The proposed "B" criteria indicate that, following significant exposure to a traumatized person, patient or client, a range of stress-related reactions (e.g., dysregulated affects, somatic symptoms, reexperience and avoidance phenomena) which were *not* present before exposure may develop.

The concept of traumatoid states includes the phenomena of vicarious traumatization as discussed by Pearlman and Saakvitne (1995) in their book, *Trauma and the Therapist*. The concept of vicarious traumatization has strong empirical support from the results of our study. The core theme of vicarious traumatization, as stated by Pearlman and Saakvitne (1995), is "the therapist that comes about as a result of empathic engagement with clients' trauma material" (p. 31). Our data strongly endorse this definition and reveal that therapists reported changes in their identity, views of society, sense of meaning in life, and disposition to prosocial advocacy on behalf of clients subsequent to their engaging in trauma work.

Our data also support the existence of transformations in the inner experiences and self-capacities of our professional participants. Moreover, the concept of vicarious traumatization fits properly within the "C" criteria proposed for traumatoid states which indicate that: "as a result of exposure to a traumatized person, alterations in psychological functioning are manifest in self-capacities, stress tolerance, world view ideologies, religious and spiritual orientation which were *not present before such exposure*." Thus, the "C" category for traumatoid states embraces a wide range of psychological changes, including alterations in inner experiences and self-capacities which may be transferred by professional work with trauma clients.

Traumatoid states, as OSRS, have conceptual consistency with experimental research on stress evoked psychobiological patterns of reactivity (Bremner, 2002; Friedman, 2000; LeDoux, 1996; McEwen, 1998; Wilson, Friedman, & Lindy, 2001; Wilson & Drozdek, 2004; Wilson & Keane, 2004). As the proposed "D" criteria indicate, traumatoid states may be transient, acute (i.e., less than 3 months), chronic (i.e., more than 6 months) or episodic in nature. As such, traumatoid states reflect the processes of allostasis and allostatic load which can result in "wear and tear" on coping and adaptation. As McEwen noted, the four subtypes of allostasis include: (1) repeated hits from multiple stressors; (2) lack of stress adaptation; (3) prolonged stressor exposure (i.e., duration); and (4) inadequate response of stress adaptation systems in the body and brain. These four types of allostasis as psychobiological processes are similar to the acute, chronic, transient and episodic nature of traumatoid states. In other words, they are neither "all or none" pheonomena nor are they necessarily pathogenic in nature. However, as the proposed "E" criteria indicate traumatoid states may vary in severity and have the potential to cause clinically significant impairment or distress in social, occupational or other areas of importance. These "E" criteria are, of course, the same as those employed in the DSM-IV for all disordered syndromes or mental disorders.

In conclusion, we suggest that the term traumatoid states, as a manifestation of OSRS, is parsimonious and integrative in nature. It incorporates the phenomena of compassion fatigue, secondary traumatic stress reactions and vicarious traumatization, but without the logical and theoretical difficulties entailed in validating secondary traumatic stress (STS or STSD) as "nearly identical" to PTSD. Indeed, neither clinical theory nor the results of our questionnaire study with all its limitations nor experimental research on allostasis support the existence of a state of stress "nearly identical" to PTSD. However, by utilizing a broader, more generic and more scientifically operational term such as traumatoid states, a wide range of seemingly diverse reactions to work with trauma clients falls neatly together under one roof and provides room for understanding in a new light the significance of trauma work in all its varied guises.

REFERENCES

Bremner, J. D. (2002). *Does stress damage the brain?* New York: Norton.

Dalenberg, C. (2000). *Countertransference and PTSD*. Washington, DC: American Psychological Association Press.

Dalenberg, C. L. (2000). *Countertransference in the treatment of trauma*. Washington, DC: American Psychological Association Press.

Derogatis, L. (1975). *Brief Symptom Inventory*. Baltimore: Clinical Psychometric Research.

Figley, C. R. (1995). *Compassion fatigue*. New York: Brunner/Mazel.

Figley, C. R. (2002). *Treating compassion fatigue*. New York: Brunner-Routledge.

Friedman, M. J. (2000). *Posttraumatic and acute stress disorders*. Kansas City, MO: Compact Clinicals.

Hedges, L. (1992). *Interpreting countertransference*. Hillsdale, NJ: Jason Aronson.

Herman, J. (1992). *Trauma and recovery*. New York: Basic Books.

Herman, J. L. (1993). Sequelae of prolonged and repeated trauma: Evidence for a complex posttraumatic syndrome (DESNOS). In J. R. T. Davidson & E. D. Foas (Eds.), *Post traumatic stress disorder: DSM–IV and beyond* (pp. 213–299). Washington, DC: American Psychiatric Press.

LeDoux, J. E. (1996). *The emotional brain*. New York: Simon & Schuster.

Maroda, K. J. (1991). *The power of countertransference*. New York: Wiley.

McEwen, B. (1998). Protective and damaging effects of stress mediators. *Seminars of the Beth Israel Deaconess Medical Center, 338*(3), 171–179.

Meldrum, L., King, R. & Spooner, D. (2002). Secondary traumatic stress in case managers working in community mental health services. In C. R. Figley (Ed.), *Treating compassion fatigue*. New York: Brunner-Routledge.

Meyers, T. W. & Cornille, T. A. (2002). The trauma of working with traumatized children. In C. R. Figley (Ed.), *Treating compassion fatigue* (pp. 39–57). New York: Brunner-Routledge.

Pearlman, L. & Saakvitne, K. (1995). *Trauma and the therapist*. New York: Norton.

Schore, A. N. (2003). *Affect regulation and the repair of the self*. New York: Norton.

Slatker, E. (1987). *Countertransference.* Northvale, NJ: Jason Aronson.

Stamm, B. H. (1995). *Secondary traumatic stress.* Lutherville, MD: Sidran Press.

Stamm, B. H. (2002). Measuring compassion satisfaction as well as fatigue: Developmental history of the compassion satisfaction and fatigue test. In C. R. Figley (Ed.), *Treating compassion fatigue.* New York: Brunner-Routledge.

Thomas, R. B. (1998). *An investigation of empathic stress reactions among mental health professionals working with PTSD.* Unpublished doctoral dissertation, Union Institute, Cincinnati, OH.

Wee, D. F. & Meyers, D. (2002). Stress responses of mental health workers following disaster: The Oklahoma City bombing. In C. R. Figley (Ed.), *Treating compassion fatigue.* New York: Brunner-Routledge.

Weiss, D. (1997). Structural clinical interview techniques. In. J. P. Wilson & T. M. Keane (Eds.), *Assessing psychological trauma and PTSD.* New York: Guilford Publications.

Weiss, D. (2004). The Impact of Events Scale—Revised. In J. P. Wilson & T. M. Keane (Eds.), *Assessing psychological trauma and PTSD* (2nd ed., pp. 425–435). New York: Guilford Publications.

Wilson, J. P. & Drozdek, B. (2004). *Broken spirits: The treatment of traumatized asylum seekers, refugees and war and torture victims.* New York: Brunner-Routledge.

Wilson, J. P. Friedman, M. J. & Lindy, J. D. (2001). *Treating psychological trauma and PTSD.* New York: Guilford Publications.

Wilson, J. P. & Keane, T. M. (Eds.). (1997). *Assisting psychological trauma and PTSD.* New York: Guilford Publications.

Wilson, J. P. & Keane, T. M. (2004). *Assessing psychological trauma and PTSD* (2nd ed.). New York: Guilford Publications.

Wolstein, B. (1988). *Essential paper on countertransference.* New York: New York University Press.

11

The Positive Therapeutic Effects of Empathic Attunement and the Transformation of Trauma

EMPATHIC ATTUNEMENT AND ALLOSTATIC TRANSFORMATIONS IN PTSD

At the heart of states of traumatization are dysregulations in organismic functioning. Trauma's impact on the wholeness, intactness and synchronized regularity of psychological functioning is altered in multileveled ways, affecting some systems of functioning more severely than others. Like a meteoroid crashing into the planet, the impact of trauma may be slight or massive. Massive traumatic impact generates changes at the surface and the depth of functioning, from the outer skin of the body to the inner neurons of the brain. Once impacted, traumatic reverberations bounce back from the brain to the external world in the form of emotion and action.

Organismic dysregulations include altered systems of adaptation: stress response systems and their interconnection with physiological systems—cardiovascular, neurohormonal, endocrine, gastrointestinal and psychological processes involving higher order cognitive processes. The exquisitely fine tuned apparatus of the human organism is altered by trauma and the resultant states of traumatization. Recovery and healing from states of traumatization involves restoring organismic fine-tuning, recalibrating stress response systems, resetting the homeostatic level of optimal system functioning, reconnecting and reintegrating previously dysregulated engineering systems governing the psychobiological basis of optimal functioning (Friedman, 2000; McEwen, 1998). Ultimately, recovery from trauma is about self-transformation and restoring meaning and wholeness to personality.

POST-TRAUMATIC STRESS DISORDER AS A DYSREGULATED PSYCHOBIOLOGICAL SYSTEM

Research, conducted by Bruce W. McEwen (1998) and his associates, has documented the nature of allostatic processes in animals and humans.

Allostasis, in brief, refers to efforts to achieve stability in levels of functioning, following changes produced by stress. Allostasis, unlike homeostasis, is a new "set point" of baseline functioning and a new level of system regulation. This new baseline set point is a different level of system function, following trauma. The organism responds to trauma with an array of defenses, protective reactions and adaptive systems which switch into higher order functioning to meet the fresh and often unexpected demands caused by traumatic injury or impact to the body and emotional systems (LeDoux, 1996). But how do states of prolonged stress response get transformed into more optimal forms of functioning? In order to answer this question, it is necessary to know how negative allostasis states get transformed into positive states.

McEwen (1998) has identified four distinct forms of allostatic load: (1) *repeated hits* from multiple stressor episodes which activate and deactivate stress response capacities; (2) *prolonged stress response* in which the stressor singly repetitiously, or multiply chronically, taxes the organism to respond with adaptive, defensive and protective measures; (3) *lack of adaptation response* which occurs when the adaptive capacity of the stress response system begins to wear down; and (4) *inadequate response* which refers to system failure, in which the psychobiologically governed engineering systems fail to perform their pre-programmed and genetically designed functions. As an example, McEwen (1998) states that, in terms of the HPA-axis of stress reactions, there "is inadequate secretion of glucocortoids, resulting in increased contributions of glucocorticoids" (p. 174). These four types of allostatic load also characterize the nature of traumatic events and the characteristics of post-traumatic stress disorder: a prolonged stress response pattern which causes impairments in adaptive functioning.

In this sense, it is possible to think of PTSD as a dysregulated psychobiological state and a form of complex allostasis. Wilson, Friedman, and Lindy (2001) have described PTSD in terms of allostatic load and identified eight distinct but interrelated patterns which characterize the complexity of prolonged stress reactions (i.e., allostatic "recalibration" of baseline functioning). These eight patterns of allostatic load processes are important to understand in terms of their capacity to be transformed through treatment. It will become apparent from the discussion in this chapter that empathic attunement and "high empathic functioning" are essential to facilitate these transformations from one psychobiological state to another. This shift in allostatic "steady states" may be thought of as a change from negative allostasis to positive allostasis. PTSD is negative allostasis, characterized by dysregulated affective, cognitive and interpersonal systems of functioning which Wilson, Friedman, and Lindy (2001) have detailed in a tetrahedral model of five sets of symptom clusters not present before the traumatic event: (i) traumatic memory and

PTSD as Allostatic Process: Dysregulated Psychobiological Systems	Empathic Attunement and Positive Allostatic Change: Organismic Tuning
1. Altered Threshold of Response Readiness to Respond Increased Levels of Hyperarousal Altered Appraisal Processes Sensitivity Threshold	**1. Stabilized Threshold of Response** Equilibrium, Steady State Functioning Decreased Levels of Hyperarousal Accurate Appraisal Processes Recalibrate Sensory Threshold
2. Hyperreactivity: Allostatic Dysregulation Inability to Modulate Arousal and Affect Alternation in Hyperarousal States Fatigue as Product of Hyperarousal	**2. Normal Psychobiological Reactivity** Ability to Modulate Affect and Arousal Affective Stability Directed, Adaptive Energy
3. Altered Initial Response Pattern Decreased Capacity for Self-Monitoring PTSD as Filter of Cognition-Perception Individual Subjective Perception of Vulnerability Altered Capacity for Self-Monitoring	**3. Stabilized Initial Response Patterns** Increased Capacity for Self-Monitoring Good Reality Testing Unfiltered by PTSD Subjective Perception of Efficacy and Coping Good Self-Monitoring
4. Altered Capacity for Internal Monitoring Decreased Capacity for Self-Monitoring Increased Risk of Misreading Internal & External Cues	**4. Good Capacity for Internal Monitoring** Increased Capacity for Self-Monitoring Decreased Risk of Misreading Cues
5. Altered Feedback Based on Distorted Information Decreased Capacity for Accurate Monitoring of Interpersonal Events Altered Cognitive Schemas Augmented or Reduced Sensory-Perceptual Modalities Proneness to Dissociation	**5. Integrative Feedback Based on Accurate Interaction** Increased Capacity for Good Interpersonal Reactions Flexible, Adaptive, Cognitive Schemas Accurate Use of Perceptual-Sensory Processes Integration in Identity Processes
6. Altered Continuous Response Increased Proneness to Avoidance Dissociation Altered Executive Functions Continuity and Flow of Behavior Disrupted	**6. Continuity in Flow of Behavior** Decreased Proneness to Dissociation Good Executive and Intellectual Functioning Continuity, Flow and Goal Directed Motivation
7. Failure to Habituate: System Failure Continued Allostasis, Nonhabituation Increased Reexperiencing Failure of System to "Shut Down"	**7. System Habituation** Habituation of Stress Response Decreased Reexperience Phenomena Adaptive System Response
8. New Allostatic Set Point Organism Recalibrates New Set Point of Adaptive Functioning	**8. New Allostatic Set Point** Return to Normal Homeostatic Functioning Different from Pretrauma Baseline

Figure 11.1 Empathic attunement and positive allostatic transformation in post-traumatic stress disorder. Copyright John P. Wilson, 2003.

reexperiencing; (ii) avoidance and numbing responses; (iii) psycho-biological changes; (iv) ego-identity and self-capacities; and (v) interpersonal relations. Figure 11.1 shows the relationship of empathic attunement and positive allostatic transformations in PTSD which will be discussed later.

TRANSFORMATION OF NEGATIVE ALLOSTATIC PROCESSES IN PTSD TO POSITIVE ALLOSTATIC STATES

To facilitate clarity in our discussion of the transformations of negative allostatic processes in PTSD to positive allostatic states, we will discuss each of the eight forms of allostatic mechanisms which are part of the complex system dynamics in PTSD. First, we will briefly discuss *negative* allostatic processes and their transformation into *positive* allostatic states. Then we will focus on the central role of empathic attunement and "high empathic functioning" in relation to the processes by which these transformations occur, that is, from one dynamic state dependent system to another more stable and enduring psychological state with normalized homeostatic functioning.

PTSD AND NEGATIVE ALLOSTASIS

Altered Thresholds of Response

In PTSD, the *thresholds of response* are altered and are reflected in four primary ways: (1) readiness to respond with the system "primed," as if another threat is forthcoming; (2) increased hyperarousal states; (3) altered sensory-perceptual processes which include hypervigilance and rapid information processing; and (4) sensitivity threshold to cues and stimuli with relevance to the evocation of adaptive stress responses.

Hyperreactivity and Allostatic Dysregulations

Part of organismic dysregulation in PTSD is the difficulty in modulating emotional responsiveness associated with manifestations of irritability, exaggerated startle responses, proneness to aggression, hypervigilance, sleep disturbances and emotional instability in mood states (e.g., anxiety, depressive reactions, heightened arousal, agitation, etc.). Persistent hyperreactivity to the precipitant stressors, or to trauma-specific cues of a generalizable nature, may lead to states of physical exhaustion, somatic complaints (e.g., muscle tension, headaches, etc.), malaise, dysphoria and feelings of depletion and chronic fatigue.

Altered Initial Response Patterns

Allostatically dysregulated states associated with trauma include decreased capacities for accurate self-monitoring of internal psychological states (e.g., affects, acuity of perception and thoughts), and subjective feelings of vulnerability which, in turn, may activate the overuse of ego-defenses. Persistent feelings of individual subjective states of vulnerability will influence cognitive capacities associated with threat appraisal, information processing, concerns for loved ones and family members, and a disposition to engage in high risk behaviors.

Altered Capacity for Internal Monitoring

Allostatic loads may alter a range of phenomena associated with capacities for internal monitoring of psychological processes. These include inaccurate perceptions of others' motives, actions, intentions and external, environmental situations. The loss of accurate monitoring of internal states is part of the changes in information processing abilities, accurate "signal detection" and executive functions. Altered capacities for internal monitoring also include the inability and lack of appreciation of psychic numbing, emotional responsiveness and interpersonal sensitivity. Extreme forms of this phenomenon include alexithymia and blunting of emotions, and the appearance of an empty, automatic, robot-like demeanor.

Altered Feedback Based on Distorted Information

Allostatic dysregulations in PTSD influence the way in which feedback from internal or external cues are processed. In general, dysregulation results in misperceptions of others' dispositions and may lead to dissociative processes. Allen N. Schore (2003a) has described this as follows:

> It has been said that the most significant consequence of the stressors of early relational trauma is the *lack of capacity for emotional self-regulation ... expressed in the loss of ability to regulate the intensity and duration of affects ...* PTSD patients, especially when stressed, show severe *deficits in pre-attentive reception and expression of facially expressed emotions, the processing of somatic information, the communication of emotional states,* the maintaining of interactions with the social environment, the use of higher levels more efficient defenses, the *capacity to access an empathic stance.* (pp. 238 and 262, italics ours)

Thus, altered feedback states, based on distorted feedback from internal states or external situations, reflect deficits in pre-attention reception processes and those of somatic states. This loss of capacity to access an empathic stance has significance for the quality of meaningful attachments and the nature of trauma transference during treatment.

Altered Continuous Responding

Alterations in continuous response tendencies in PTSD refer to disruptions or interruptions in the "flow" of behavior, due to system dysregulation at multiple levels (i.e., by PTSD symptoms). In other words, continuous responding is correlated directly with the threshold of responsiveness in behavioral adaptation. This alteration in the continuity and flow of behavior is most evident in dissociative processes, hypervigilance states, predicaments of concentration and inattentiveness, and problem solving difficulties, particularly in the areas of emotional conflicts of an interpersonal nature.

Failure to Habituate: Stress Response System Failure

Allostatic load in the extreme results in system failure and the non-habituation of maladaptive response associated with PTSD. Wang, Wilson, and Mason (1996) characterized this as part of a downward cycle of decompensation which moves from adaptive to extremely maladaptive patterns of coping. Summarizing this research data, Allen N. Schore (2003b) says,

> [there] are incremental impairments in amplified hyperarousal systems and defensive dissociation, decreased range of spontaneity and facial expression, heightened dysregulation of self-esteem, deepening loss of contact with the environment, reduced attachment and insight, and increased probability of destruction and suicide... (p. 263)

Allostatically driven states in PTSD associated with nonhabituation indicate that the organism is in an "overdriven" state of functioning which may amplify subsystems associated with the range of PTSD behaviors. Excessive and prolonged hyperarousal states may lead to patterns of decompensation and coping described by Wang, Wilson, and Mason (1996). Persistent hyperarousal and nonhabituating stress response can effect different syndromes of behavior which include high-risk activity, sensation seeking, addictive acting out, depression, withdrawal, isolation, suicidal states, dissociative and altered ego-states (Chu, 1999; Putnam, 1997; Wang, Wilson, & Mason, 1996; Wilson, 1989; Wilson & Zigelbaum, 1986).

New Allostatic Set Point in Organismic Functioning

Allostatic loads in PTSD eventually run their course and habituate. When habituation of the prolonged stress response characteristic of PTSD occurs, a new organismic set point is established. This "recalibrated" set point is a new state of equilibrium in functioning which is different from the psychobiological organismic state that existed prior to the traumatic event. This is what McEwen (1998) meant when he characterized allostasis as attempts at stability through changed states of functioning. Like a ship that has been tossed about by powerful winds in the ocean and capsizes, it will eventually right itself or sink.

We can regard organismic "tuning" as a set of processes by which negative allostatic processes are transformed into positive allostatic reconfigurations of organismic functioning. Recovery and healing from PTSD is positive allostatic functioning at all levels of integrated organismic functioning.

POSITIVE ALLOSTATIC TRANSFORMATIONS IN PTSD AND TRAUMA-RELATED CONDITIONS

Figure 11.1 summarizes the characteristics of positive allostatic transformation in PTSD which occur with effective treatments (see Foa, Keane, & Friedman, 2001; Wilson, Friedman, & Lindy, 2001, for a discussion of effective PTSD treatments). We will discuss how each of the negative allostatic processes is transformed through effective treatment modalities of PTSD and then discuss the role of empathic attunement and "high empathic functioning" in those processes. Note that our discussion does not cover particular therapeutic approaches to PTSD treatment (e.g., cognitive-behavioral, psychoanalytic, pharmacological, EMDR, etc.) but focuses instead on the resultant changes in organismic functioning.

Stabilized Thresholds of Response

Transformation of negative allostatic states into positive ones results in a stabilized threshold of response. This includes equilibrium and steady state functioning, rather than dysregulated affects and hyperarousal conditions which decrease and return to a new homeostatic baseline. Sensitivity thresholds in sensory-perceptual processes regain their acuity and accuracy in function, leading to realistic (i.e., accurate) appraisal processes of environmental cues.

Normal Psychobiological Reactivity

Positive allostasis reflects normal and usually optimal levels of psychobiological reactivity, characterized by the ability to modulate affect and arousal, and involves emotional stability in interpersonal transactions. Subjectively, PTSD clients are aware of the positive change in their organismic state; describe it using words like "calmness," "relaxed," "quiescent," "normal," "no longer wired up, edgy, tense, or on guard," and feel more comfortable with continuity in responding to disruptions, previously caused by intrusive PTSD processes, and the need for security and defense measures to protect states of inner vulnerability.

Stabilized Initial Response Patterns

Positive allostasis restores the capacity for good self-monitoring of inner processes and more accurate person perception, reality testing and "signal detection" of environmental cues, achieving a subjective sense of efficacy in coping. PTSD clients feel more in control of themselves and find increased ability to accurately monitor their formerly hyperaroused states, reinforcing their efforts towards mastery, achievement and enjoyment of self-chosen pursuits.

Good Capacity for Self-Monitoring

Positive allostasis results in better cognitive processing at all levels of functioning. The encoding, processing and storage of information is more efficient and productive, and the capacity to accurately read internal and external cues is improved. Sensory-perceptual processes are no longer subject to distortions due to trauma specific cues (TSCs; Wilson & Lindy, 1994) associated with trauma related learning and produced by classical or operant conditioning. The behavioral and interpersonal consequences associated with misreading cues are substantially diminished, but can be reactivated by episodes of reexperiencing phenomena triggered by TSCs or more common forms of stimulus generalization. The psychobiological engineering systems that were rendered insufficient or maladaptive are restored to their pre-programmed genetic functions without any interfering "noise" caused by PTSD symptoms.

Integrative Use of Feedback Based on Accurate Information

Organismic tuning, through positive allostatic transformations, enables the integrative use of feedback based on accurate information which stems from cognitive-perceptual processes and increased executive functions of the intellect. The PTSD client, through subjective feelings of efficacy or good capacity to modulate affect and profoundly altered (i.e., reduced) states of hyperarousal, can now integrate feedback into memory and repertoires of instrumental coping. As a consequence, the PTSD patient manifests more flexibility in cognitive schemas and greater ability to problem solve and find answers to everyday difficulties without anxiety, states of vulnerability, fear, anger or frustration. This increased capacity to integrate information into right and left hemisphere brain functions is experienced as comfort since dysregulated affects no longer impair right brain activity (Schore, 2003b).

Continuity in the Flow of Behavior

Positive allostasis leads to the restoration of continuity in the flow of behavior. The resolution and/or reduction of hyperarousal states characteristic of PTSD reduces stress symptoms. It decreases the defensive need to ward off anxiety; protect against and avoid distressing reexperiences of trauma; and to suffer from disrupted regulatory behaviors, such as sleeping, eating and coping with everyday stressors. Continuity in the flow of behavior also refers to psychoformative developments (Lifton, 1976) which indicate a sense of connection, growth and integration in self-processes. The hyperaroused, overly anxious or numbed self now feels an inner sense of aliveness, animation, direction and capacity to envision the self-in-the-future. The subjective experience of flow and continuity in the post-traumatically transformed self is a manifestation of high energy, creativity and enhanced feelings of well-being. In some cases, especially in survivors of belief-shattering encounters which challenge the meaning of life at the most existential level, a sense of flow and continuity may be felt as the rebirth of the soul, since continuity with past history had been destroyed.

System Habituation

In positive allostasis, the prolonged stress response inherent in PTSD habituates; the triad of core PTSD symptom clusters (i.e., reexperience, avoidance, hyperarousal) attenuate in severity, frequency and duration. New adaptive stress responses replace "overdriven" states of organismic functioning (Schore, 2003b). Organismic tuning means that maladaptive forms of stress response, reflective of severe "wear and tear," are repaired and recalibrated to be finely tuned, permitting optimal states of functioning without pathological consequences to psychosocial behavior, epigenetic and life course development. The transformation of negative allostatic pathological states to positive, nonpathological states results in new allostasis set points, with altered but stabilized baselines reflective of a genuine capacity for adaptation and growth.

New Allostatic Set Points: Optimal Positive State Potential

The transformation of negative allostasis in PTSD to positive allostasis mirrors a change in organismic states from traumatization to the potential for optimal growth and psychosocial functioning. Positive allostasis is the gradual return to homeostasis, equilibrium and the capacity to regulate affect dysregulation. It occurs at multiple levels of psychological functioning since the organism itself is holistic and integrated in nature (Miller, 1978).

Wilson, Friedman and Lindy (2001), in a review of the treatment approaches for PTSD and their goals, summarize the objectives of post-traumatic therapies as follows: (1) the reestablishment of normal stress response patterns; (2) the facilitation of normalization towards homeostasis by medication; (3) the restoration towards normal intrapsychic functioning and the reduction in need for maladaptive ego-defenses; (4) the establishment of authority and controls over traumatic memories; (5) the restoration of positive self-capacities; (6) the restoration of healthy epigenetic and life span development; and (7) the fostering of recovery within an embedded cultural framework. These treatment goals are indicative of positive allostatic changes in organismic functioning and, as such, reflect new levels of stability through changes in coping, adaptation and ego-mastery.

Post-traumatic therapies utilize different techniques to assist victims of trauma in recovery. For example, pharmacotherapy strives to reduce psychological states of anxiety, depression and anxiety; cognitive behavioral treatment seeks the reordering of distorted frames of thinking and overwhelming traumatic memories; and psychoanalytical methods identify and interpret maladaptive defenses. However, the success of any therapeutic approach requires an understanding of how individuals are uniquely traumatized by their experiences. Understanding the inner experience of traumatization presupposes accurate knowledge gained through the process of empathy and empathic attunement. The question then arises as to how empathic attunement facilitates organismic tuning.

THE TRANSMITTING UNCONSCIOUS OF TRAUMATIZATION REVISITED

Empathy, Signal Processing and Affect Modulation: Isochronicity and Dyschronicity in Treatment

In chapter 1, we described the nature of multichanneled information transmission by the patient to the therapist in the course of treatment. These seven channels (affects, defense, somatic states, ego states, personality, unconscious memory and cognitive-perceptual processes) organismically embed the patient's trauma experience. During treatment, trauma transference (TST) occurs through these seven channels in varying degrees of frequency, duration, amplitude and intensity. This variability in transmission by the different organismic channels reflects allostatic states, in the way a computer's central processing unit "flickers" in response to iconic activity on a monitor screen, indicating the degrees of internal activity operating at any given time. In the course of treatment (i.e., beginning, middle and end), the information flow from the patient to the therapist will show variability of type *within and between* the seven channels of signal transmissions of organismic states. As movement towards integration occurs, the channels synchronize, showing similarity in styles, and reflecting more integrated levels of organismic functioning. On the other hand, extreme fragmentation of the self caused by trauma will be manifest in dysynchronous patterns and marked variability in the signal transmissions, showing patterns that "crisscross" rather than flow isomorphically with each other in a smooth, synchronous way. Indeed, the greater the degree of post-traumatic pathology, the greater the degree of affect dysregulation and unconscious motivational power and the demand for cognitive-perceptual energies associated with internal processing requirements. In extreme trauma related psychopathology, the multichanneled signal transmissions are noisy and contain confusing, conflicting and "hidden" signal transmissions among themselves. For example, this pattern is clearly evident in dissociative identity disorder, where a new "alter" personality emerges and presents itself to the therapist as part of a much larger constellation of personality organization. Similarly, multichanneled signal transmissions can be observed in dissociative "flashback" states, where a patient is suddenly flooded with visual images and emotionally reexperiences the overwhelming nature of a trauma.

To the therapist or observer, the sudden and dramatic change in behavior is evident, and it is apparent that the patient is "back there again," reexperiencing with strong emotion what was traumatically stressful in vivid ways. In contrast, however, any of the seven channels in states of psychic numbing can undergo disruptions in the clarity of signal transmissions which suppress variability in signal modulations in an attempt to maintain a sense of internal control over feared affects and traumatic memories. Psychic numbing is a manifestation of strongly overregulated signal transmissions which, paradoxically, result in "messages" of the degree of defensively contained dysregulated affect. The degree of psychic numbing is directly related to the degree of internal fears of vulnerability—fears of expressing emotions, guilt and information about what occurred during the trauma, lest such disclosure results in de-compensation, total affect dysregulation and cathartic discharge, overwhelming and uncontrollable anxiety states, or annihilation of the self and personal identity. In the most extreme cases of psychic numbing, the patient fears that to let go of overcontrolled states of numbing will culminate in death or self-destruction.

PATTERNS OF ISOCHRONICITY AND DYSCHRONICITY BETWEEN PATIENT AND THERAPIST DURING TREATMENT

Figure 11.2 illustrates the relationship between empathy, signal processing, affect modulation and states of isochronicity and dyschronicity between the patient and the therapist during treatment.

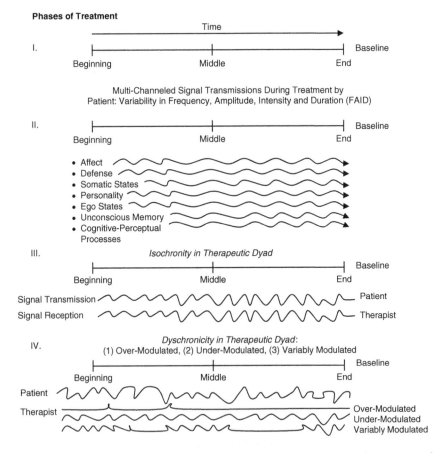

Figure 11.2 Empathy, signal processing and affect modulation: Isochronicity and dyschronicity in treatment. Copyright John P. Wilson, 2003.

Baseline Functioning in Phases of Treatment

To begin, Figure 11.2 shows a chronological time line of treatment: beginning, middle and end phases (see I). This is a simplification to represent a baseline of the patient's functioning in terms of post-traumatic symptoms of behavior patterns.

Multichannel Signal Transmissions in Post-traumatic Therapy

The second illustration (II) shows the signal transmissions in seven channels (affects, defence, somatic states, ego-states, personality, unconscious memory, cognitive-perceptual processes) across time intervals in treatment. The signal transmissions reflect organismic states of being at any given point in time. The transmissions can be construed in many ways: waves, flow, energy, affects, data, information, encapsulated signal data, and so forth. As such, the transmissions reflect embedded allostatic organismic processes which are sent from the patient to the therapist by trauma transference.

Isochronicity in Therapeutic Dyad

Isochronicity in the therapeutic dyad is represented in the third illustration (III). In isochronicity, the therapist maintains empathic attunement and congruency in responding. The therapist accurately tracks and decodes signal transmissions from the patient in the seven channels. As a result, a concordance and isochronous pattern exists in the therapeutic dyad, as shown in III. However, isochronicity in the therapist's response does not mean that the therapist empathically experiences the same level of organismic dysregulation as the patient. Rather, the therapist accurately monitors, understands and acquires knowledge of the patient's internal psychological states and communicates this understanding in an isochronous way, with proper cadence, timing, resonance and interpretation in the communication flow of information between them.

Dyschronicity in Therapeutic Dyad

Dyschronicity in the therapeutic dyad is illustrated in IV, showing three forms of dyschronous states: (1) overmodulated, (2) undermodulated, and (3) variably modulated. The degrees of deviation from isochronicity determine: (1) overmodulated, (2) undermodulated, or (3) variably modulated states in the therapist.

Overmodulated Dyschronous States

The classic example of overmodulation is the excessive reliance on the "blank screen" therapeutic façade or the obsessively rigid adherence to analytic protocol (Wolstein, 1988). In either case, the overmodulated therapeutic stance is not isochronously in synchronization with the patient and fails to communicate a clear, unambiguous sense of reception and processing of what was transmitted by the patient in *some or all* of the seven channels of organismic transmission.

Undermodulated Dyschronous States

In undermodulated dyschronous states, the therapistsuffers a consistent inability to maintain stability, affect modulation and isochronicity in responding to the client. The therapist manifests undermodulated states and deviates, in smaller or larger degrees, in the capacity to accurately track, decode and interpret organismic signal transmissions. In this sense, the therapist never "connects," "clicks," and "meets the patient with empathic equality" during the course of treatment.

Variably Modulated Dyschronous States

In variably modulated states, the therapist goes through conspicuous alternating patterns of overmodulated and undermodulated states. This tendency towards cyclical alternation between overmodulated and undermodulated states in the therapist reflects allostasis, empathic strains and Type I and Type II countertransference. Variable modulation results in fluctuation in the degree of accurate tracking, decoding and interpretation of signal transmissions from the patient. Variably modulated states are "hit and miss," sometimes "on target," through empathic attunement and, at other times, "off target" and out of range. Variably modulated states are directly associated with empathic strain and allostatic load in the therapist. In more severe cases of dyschronicity, the resultant inconsistency is a potential manifestation of a traumatoid condition in the therapist, which may require supervision, analysis or educational consultation.

ORGANISMIC TUNING: THE POSITIVE THERAPEUTIC EFFECTS OF EMPATHIC ATTUNEMENT

Our analysis of the effects of empathic attunement in the treatment of psychological trauma and PTSD emphasizes that phasic synchrony is a process associated with natural healing. We are using the term *natural healing* to describe positive allostatic readjustment following trauma; a recalibration of the organisms adaptation to stress and movement towards a resolution of the unmetabolized psychic elements of the trauma experience (Wilson & Lindy, 1994). Positive allostasis is restabilization following change; a reorganization of the organism following the fragmenting impact of trauma. The configuration of organismic restructuring as positive allostasis has many variations which range on a continuum from minimal to radical transformation of the self and manifestations in behavior.

However, it must be recognized that currently we have no classification system for the phases, forms or patterns of personality transformations that occur as part of positive allostatic reorganization. Neither do we have a reference handbook of post-traumatic self-integration which classifies forms of healthy personality emerging beyond the pathology of PTSD and its co-morbidities. Considered in a broader perspective, we do not yet understand the positive organismic sources associated with resiliency, a sense of coherency and transformative integration of ego-space and the structure of the self (Wilson, 2004; Wilson & Drozdek, 2004).

A shift of focus now allows us to examine the manner in which empathic accuracy, as a qualitative phenomenon, relates to the successful treatment of psychological trauma and PTSD. Figure 11.3 summarizes 15 points for understanding the means whereby empathic congruence, phasic synchrony and isochronicity facilitate the mechanisms of allostatic transformations from negative to positive in nature.

---

1. Empathy and the Quantity of Information
2. Empathy and the Quality of Information
3. Trauma Linkage: Coupling the Elements Together
4. The Gestalt of Trauma
5. Precision and Accuracy of Decoding Trauma Specific Information
6. The Role of Empathy in Informational Density and Cognitive Complexity
7. Empathy and Portals of Entry to Ego-Space Configuration
8. Trauma Disclosure and Reduction in Defensiveness
9. Clarity in Understanding: Ego-Defenses Built around Traumatization
10. Positive Allostasis: Restabilization following Change Caused by Trauma
11. Threshold of TST Recognition and Utilization in Treatment
12. Symbolization of Trauma Experience
13. Empathy and Information Storage: Future Stockpiles
14. Individual Therapist Awareness of Empathic Strain, Compassion Fatigue and Countertransference Processes
15. Isochronicity and Organismic Tuning:Holistic Healing through Positive Allostatic Restabilization

---

Figure 11.3 Isochronicity and organismic tuning: The positive therapeutic effects of empathic attunement. Copyright John P. Wilson, 2002.

EMPATHY AND THE TRANSFORMATION OF TRAUMA AND PTSD

Empathy and the Quantity of Information

Empathic congruence leads to the disclosure of a sufficient amount of information about negative allostasis. Because of phasic synchrony and isochronicity, the establishment of empathic congruence helps patients to feel understood, secure and desirous of explaining how they have changed and been affected by the traumatic experience.

Empathy and the Quality of Information

By definition, phasic synchrony and empathic attunement with good resonance (precision) generates accurate information flow from the patient. The therapist's ability to stay phasically synchronized enhances the quality and detail of information about the trauma experience and its impact on the existing personality dynamics and history of the patient.

Trauma Linkage: Coupling the Trauma Elements Together

Empathic attunement facilitates the therapist's ability to make the necessary links in the reconstruction of the patient's trauma history. Trauma linkage means that both the therapist and the patient can discover how the magnitude of trauma restructured the organism, altering the configuration of ego-space and the constellation of self-processes. Establishing trauma links to the various elements of the allostatic changes wrought by the trauma enables discovery of how the trauma complex was formed (Wilson, 2003). In this way, both patient and therapist can "see" the entire picture of the trauma's impact in a manner similar to a viewing together of an xray, MRI or PET scan of the body or brain. More specifically, once the structure of the trauma complex is evident, the process of therapy becomes analogous to having a functional MRI image in real time for understanding organismic functioning in a holistic manner. In other words, the dynamics of the process become transparent.

The Gestalt of Trauma

The establishment of linkages in the trauma complex facilitates understanding the *Gestalt of Trauma* in the patient's life. The gestalt of trauma signifies the ability to fit all of the pieces of the puzzle together; to see the whole constellation, as well as the individual parts, in a manner not evident in their original state, following the changes produced by the traumatic impact.

Precision and Accuracy in Decoding Trauma Specific Information

Empathic attunement is synonymous with precision and accuracy in responding to the patient. Empathic congruence and phasic synchrony in therapeutic orientation enables the decoding of TST and the unconscious transmission of "leaked" information which the patient wishes to convey but may not be able to verbalize (see chapter 1). Unconscious transmissions, especially in nonverbal body posture or somatic complaints, may represent condensed symbolic material with multiple meanings which have been warded off by defenses or transformed into symbolized communications.

The Role of Empathy in Informational Density and Cognitive Complexity

The treatment of trauma and PTSD is a dynamic, dual unfolding process of transference and countertransference. The patient and the therapist have reciprocal effects on each other during the course of treatment. They are like fellow sojourners on a trip that exposes them to the unknown and, at times, the frightening chasm of psychic uncertainty. However, the capacity for sustained empathic attunement yields changes in the therapist's cognitive processes: (a) information density, and (b) cognitive complexity, which are related by-products of the encoding knowledge about the patient's psychodynamics (Aronoff & Wilson, 1985). Information density connotes the amount (density) of the elements configured in the ego-space of the patient's trauma complex (Wilson, 2003), and cognitive complexity refers to organizational differentiation of that material in the therapist's cognitive schema. Empathic accuracy facilitates greater cognitive complexity of information processing by the therapist.

Empathy and Portals of Entry to Ego-Space Configuration

Empathic attunement enables the therapist to identify more easily the various portals of entry into the patient's ego-space and the nexus of the trauma complex and PTSD. Wilson, Friedman, and Lindy (2001) have identified five portals of access to the interior sanctum of PTSD processes—the five clusters of PTSD symptom configuration. The creative therapist who is empathically attuned can enter these portals as avenues for gaining more information on the manner in which the patient is processing the traumatic experience. Trauma alters the organisms in synergistic ways—some subtle, and others intricately complicated. Further, one implication of phasic synchrony is the ability to resonate with the organismic expressions of traumatic impacts, for example, with ego-defenses and areas of emotional vulnerability and injury; with physiological hyperreactivity, dreams, affective lability, resistances, and areas of avoidance, denial, dissociation, disavowal and numbing. Since PTSD symptoms are transduced into seven channels of symptom transmission, access to the portals of entry into the patient's ego-space is like walking down a dark passageway into various chambers hidden by the façade of the patient's persona. Empathic congruence becomes a beacon of light which illuminates the pathways, focusing light in the necessary areas to properly traverse the hallway into the hidden chambers of the unconscious.

Trauma Disclosure and Reduction of Defensiveness

Entry into the patient's ego-space via empathic congruence and the mechanisms of phasic synchrony facilitates a more complete disclosure of the contents of the trauma narrative by the patient. This process of disclosure will, over time, result in a reduction in the need for defensive guardedness and protection. Genuine empathic attunement conveys the message from therapists that they, as the source of comfort and safety, protect patients from their fears and anxieties associated with organismic disequilibrium which result from allostatic changes in the pretrauma baseline of functioning.

Clarity in Understanding Ego-Defenses Built around Traumatization

As a corollary to increased trauma disclosure and reduction of defensiveness in the patient, the therapist develops understanding of the role of ego-defenses in protecting areas of vulnerability associated with traumatization. Authentic empathic attunement is one form of what Carl Rogers (1951) termed *unconditional positive regard for the patient*. The process of sustained authentic attunement gives the therapist a broader vista of the operation of the patient's defenses, the need for which, paradoxically, lessens in the context of a therapeutic sanctuary which the patient can experience as a place of rock solid safety amidst the inner turmoil of uncertainty and the search for meaning and purpose to individual trauma experiences.

Threshold of TST Recognition and Utilization in Treatment

The therapist's capacity to recognize and properly utilize TST varies greatly in the treatment of PTSD. Empathic congruence and phasic synchrony facilitates the achievement of a higher threshold of recognition of TST, enabling the therapist to quickly recognize and use this form of transference in the treatment process. As stated earlier, TST is considered to be present throughout the course of treatment, and therefore empathic attunement enables recognition of its transmissions, dynamic significance and critical importance as information "leakage" from patient to therapist (see chapters 1 and 4).

Symbolization of Trauma Experience

The capacity of humans to symbolize experience has long been recognized in the psychodynamic literature (Freud, 1917; Jung, 1929; Lindy, 1993). Traumatic experiences, as archetypal phenomena, are also symbolized to express the patient's intrapsychic processes (Early, 1993; Kalsched, 1996). Empathic accuracy serves as a vehicle by which to understand the idiosyncratic manifestation of the trauma experience. The symbolization of the trauma experience is yet another variation of "information transmission" from patients. It is their way of saying, "Look at this symbol; it contains representations of how I was affected by trauma; it is a clue for you to understand that which I cannot fully verbalize." We can also regard symbols of trauma as encapsulated information containing categories of data which link elements of the trauma experience together in a unified manner. The symbols are generated by the patient's "unconscious architect" who creates an object of expression. Interpretation of, or understanding its meaning, may be obscured from the patient's conscious awareness but, of course, may be unconsciously informative when accurately interpreted.

Empathy and Information Storage: Future Stockpiles

Empathic accuracy and congruence are associated with the capacity to receive, decode and use information generated by the patient. In addition to the quantity and quality of information retrieved through the patient's multichanneled transmissions, such data can be stored by the therapist for future use in formulating the nature of psychodynamic functioning. Clearly, having more information about the patient is critically important in several ways: first, to formulate hypotheses about the operation of allostatic mechanisms in PTSD and associated co-morbidities; second, to use the stored information as an additional tool of sustained empathic attunement, including, for example, hypothesis testing with patients about their functioning; third, to increase prediction through empathic accuracy, i.e., to anticipate patterns of behavior likely to be expressed by the patient in the course of "working through" the trauma (assimilation and accommodation of unmetabolized traumatic material).

Increased Therapist Awareness of Empathic Strain, Traumatoid States and Countertransference Processes

As a natural consequence of sustained empathic attunement, empathic congruence, matching phenomena, etc., therapists develop greater self-awareness and insight into their own reactions to the work of treatment. Clearly, good empathic capacity implies awareness not only of the patient's internal psychological state, but also of the therapist's internal affective and psychological processes. Thus, self-directed empathic intro-spection (i.e., self-monitoring) is a mode through which analysts identify their own reactions indicative of empathic strains, traumatoid states and countertransference processes.

Isochronicity and Organismic Tuning: Holistic Healing Through Positive Allostatic Restabilization

Organismic tuning refers to positive allostatic readjustment following a traumatic experience. Positive allostasis denotes restabilization in a holis-tic way that promotes growth, resilience and efficacious functioning rather than stasis, fixation, fragmentation and maladaptive psycho-pathology. Organismic tuning, or isochronicity, is a natural consequence of consistent, sustained, empathic inquiry. Organismic tuning also reflects holistic, synergistic interactive effects in the psychobiology of human stress response (Friedman, 2000). Sustained, consistent, empathic congruence which accurately decodes the transference and trauma specific transmissions (TSTT) of the patient facilitates positive allostatic restabilization, leading to organismic growth, health, optimal func-tioning and movement towards the increased self-actualization of potentials.

Positive Allostasis: Restabilization following Change Caused by Trauma

Empathic attunement in its various permutations also serves to facilitate positive allostasis. It is the creation of a new configuration of psychologi-cal and behavioral adaptation. As noted by Horowitz (1986), a process of accommodation occurs in handling the trauma experience: what was ego-alien (trauma) is now assimilated into a new cognitive-affective structure of ego-processes and the self. Although positive allostasis is not identical to psychological health, it is a central mechanism in the process of heal-ing. In this regard, transformation of the trauma experience into an inte-grative, efficacious self-modality, without debilitating symptoms of anxiety, depression, substance abuse, PTSD, and so on, may be regarded as the core of healing and organismic resilience.

In conclusion, it is our belief that "high empathic functioning," as described in chapter 5, is a fundamental psychological state of the therapist which facilitates positive allostasis and the transformation of negative allostatic conditions in the organism caused by trauma. High empathic functioning is optimal therapeutic efficacy and promotes growth. High empathic functioning is the ability to sense or intuit the "big picture" of the client's internal psychological state of being; to see the underlying dynamic designs, defense structures, thought patterns, dys-regulated organismic conditions at multisystem levels; and to compre-hend behavioral dispositions without imposing judgment on conditions of worth on the client. High empathy is the capacity to be fully present in-the-moment with the client in a way that facilitates the naturalistic processes of self-healing.

REFERENCES

Aronoff, J. & Wilson, J. P. (1985). *Personality in the social process*. Livingston, NJ: Erlbaum.

Chu, J. A. (1999). *Rebuilding shattered lives: The responsible treatment of complex post-traumatic and dissociative disorders*. New York: Wiley.

Early, E. (1993). *The raven's return: The influences of psychological trauma on individuals and cul-ture*. New York: Chiron Publications.

Foa, E., Keane, T. M. & Friedman, M. J. (2001). *Effective treatments for PTSD*. New York: Guilford Publications.

Freud, S. (1917a). *Introductory lecture on psychoanalysis*. New York: Norton.

Freud, S. (1917b). *New introductory lectures on psychoanalysis*. New York: Norton.

Friedman, M. J. (2000). *Posttraumatic and acute stress disorders*. Kansas City, MO: Compact Clinicals.

Horowitz, M. (1986). *Stress response syndromes* (2nd ed.). Northvale, NJ: Jason Aronson.

McCann, L. & Pearlman, L. (1990). *Psychological trauma and the adult survivor*. New York: Brunner/Mazel.

Jung, C. G. (1929). The therapeutic value of abreaction (H. Read, M. Fordham & G. Adler, Eds., Vol. 16). In *Collected works of C. J. Jung* (Vols. 1–20, R. F. C. Hull, Trans.). Princeton, NJ: Princeton University Press.

Jung, C. G. (1953–1979). *Collected works of C. G. Jung* (Vols. 1–20, R. F. C. Hull, Trans., & H. Read, M. Fordham & G. Adler, Eds.). Princeton, NJ: Princeton University Press.

Kalsched, D. (1996). *The inner world of trauma: Archetypal defenses of the personal spirit*. London: Routledge.

LeDoux, J. E. (1996). *The emotional brain*. New York: Simon & Schuster.

Lifton, R. J. (1976). *The life of the self*. New York: Simon & Schuster.

Lindy, J. D. (1993). Focal psychoanalytic psychotherapy of PTSD. In J. P. Wilson & B. Raphael (Eds.), *International handbook of traumatic stress syndromes* (pp. 803–811). New York: Plenum Press.

McEwen, B. (1998). Protective and damaging effects of stress mediators. *Seminars of the Beth Israel Deaconess Medical Center, 338*(3), 171–179.

Miller, J. G. (1978). *Living systems*. New York: McGraw-Hill.

Pearlman, L. & Saakvitne, K. (1995). *Trauma and the therapist*. New York: Norton.

Putnam, F. (1997). *Dissociation in children and adolescents*. New York: Guilford Publications.

Rogers, C. (1951). *Client centered therapy*. New York: Houghton Mifflin.

Schore, A. N. (2003a). *Affect dysregulation and repair of the self*. New York: Norton.

Schore, A. N. (2003b). *Affect regulation and the repair of the self*. New York: Norton.

Wang, S., Wilson, J. P. & Mason, J. (1996). Stages and decompensation in combat related PTSD: A new conceptual model. *Integrative Physiological and Behavioral Science, 31*(3), 236–253.

Wilson, J. P. (1989). *Trauma, transformation and healing: An integrated approach to theory, research and post-traumatic theory*. New York: Brunner/Mazel.

Wilson, J. P. (2004). PTSD and complex PTSD: Symptoms, syndromes and diagnoses. In J. P. Wilson & T. M. Keane (Eds.), *Assessing psychological trauma and PTSD* (2nd ed., pp. 1–47). New York: Guilford Publications.

Wilson, J. P. & Drozdek, B. (2004). *Broken spirits: The treatment of traumatized asylum seekers, refugees and war and torture victims*. New York: Brunner-Routledge.

Wilson, J. P., Friedman, M. J. & Lindy, J. D. (2001). *Treating psychological trauma and PTSD*. New York: Guilford Publications.

Wilson, J. & Lindy, J. (1994). *Countertransference in the treatment of PTSD*. New York: Guilford Publications.

Wilson, J. P. & Zigelbaum, S. D. (1986). PTSD and the disposition to criminal behavior. In C. R. Figley (Ed.), *Trauma and its wake* (Vol. 2, pp. 305–321). New York: Brunner/Mazel.

Appendix

CTRS®

CLINICIANS' TRAUMA REACTION SURVEY

> As a helping professional, clinician, researcher or academician, if you work with trauma clients, PTSD or allied conditions, please fill out this survey.

This survey is being conducted as a doctoral research study through *The Union Institute in Cincinnati, Ohio, by Rhiannon B. Thomas, M.S., under the supervision of John P. Wilson. Ph.D., past president of ISTSS. The goal of this study is increased understanding of the impact on helping professionals of working with traumatized clients. All surveys are anonymous and confidential.* Some respondents may find completing this survey stimulates awareness and provokes emotion about the nature of their work. Most persons typically finish within 25 minutes. Special thanks to the administrators and members of *The International Society for the Study of Dissociation (ISSD) and The International Society for Traumatic Stress Studies (ISTSS)* for their interest and cooperation in this study. Announcement of the availability of The Clinicians' Trauma Reaction Survey (CTRS) findings will be noted in the news letters of each society. If you do not work with or treat trauma related clients (PTSD and allied conditions), please pass this survey along to a colleague who does.

Thank you for your consideration, time, and assistance.

Survey Instructions

Please respond to the items provided which are reported reactions of therapists and other helping professionals who treat or work with trauma survivors in a clinical, academic, or research setting. Your responses should reflect your entire professional experience in working with trauma survivors.

- Please read each statement.
- Choose from the selections provided: (0) Never (1) Rarely (2) Sometimes (3) Often (4) Always.

- Circle the number (i.e., scale point 0-4) that best applies to you in your work with trauma survivors, reflecting your experience as a professional over the course of your career.
- Please do not place your name or any identifying information on the survey as we do not want to identify individuals. This survey is designed to be anonymous and confidential.
- Please answer the demographic questions on the back of this booklet.
- Please return your completed questionnaire to:

Instructions

Please read each statement on page 237. Circle the number that best applies to you in your work with trauma survivors from among the provided selections of:
(0) Never
(1) Rarely
(2) Sometimes
(3) Often
(4) Always

Instructions

Some professionals report changes in their outlook after working with trauma clients. Please read the following and circle the number that best applies to your experience.

	Never	Rarely	Sometimes	Often	Always	
1	0	1	2	3	4	I have felt overwhelmed by the trauma story of my client(s).
2	0	1	2	3	4	I have experienced uncertainty as to my ability to work with my trauma client(s).
3	0	1	2	3	4	I have experienced a sense of personal vulnerability while listening to the trauma story of my client(s).
4	0	1	2	3	4	I have experienced a sense of disequilibrium or "being off balance" while listening to the trauma story of my client.
5	0	1	2	3	4	I have experienced difficulty controlling my feelings, while listening to the story of my trauma client(s).
6	0	1	2	3	4	While listening to my trauma client(s), I have felt a need to hide behind a professional role.
7	0	1	2	3	4	I have experienced the need to intellectualize the trauma story in order to avoid personal distress.
8	0	1	2	3	4	While with my trauma client(s), I have found myself thinking about things unrelated to my client and their issues.
9	0	1	2	3	4	While listening to my trauma client(s), I have found my attention lapsing and my thoughts drifting.
10	0	1	2	3	4	I have felt a need to distance myself emotionally from my trauma client(s) during the session or away from the off.
11	0	1	2	3	4	While listening to my trauma client(s), I have thought about difficult emotional experiences in my own life.
12	0	1	2	3	4	I have experienced unwanted feelings and memories from my past, while listening to my trauma client(s).
13	0	1	2	3	4	I have found myself not wanting to believe the trauma story of my client(s).
14	0	1	2	3	4	I have found myself wondering why I chose to work with trauma clients.
15	0	1	2	3	4	I have become frustrated with trauma clients who are difficult to move forward.
16	0	1	2	3	4	I have wanted to exclude from my awareness the disturbing content of my client(s) trauma story.
17	0	1	2	3	4	I have experienced concerns for my trauma client(s) that extend beyond the working setting.
18	0	1	2	3	4	I have felt a strong sense of personal identification with some of my trauma client(s).
19	0	1	2	3	4	I have found it difficult to maintain firm boundaries with my trauma client(s) due to the intensity of their needs.
20	0	1	2	3	4	I have experienced a need to be an advocate for my client(s) because of the victimization they have endured.
21	0	1	2	3	4	I have found it easy to help my trauma client(s) control their feelings.
22	0	1	2	3	4	I have experienced a need to protect, rescue, or shelter my trauma client(s) from the abuses they have suffered.
23	0	1	2	3	4	I have experienced the wish that my trauma client(s) not show up for the scheduled appointments.
24	0	1	2	3	4	I have experienced emotional or empathic detachment while working with trauma clients.
25	0	1	2	3	4	I have had thoughts of referring my trauma client(s) to someone else for help.

	Never	Rarely	Sometimes	Often	Always	
26	0	1	2	3	4	There have been times when I have wished that I did not have to work with trauma client(s).
27	0	1	2	3	4	I have purposely canceled appointments to avoid dealing with my trauma client(s).
28	0	1	2	3	4	I have experienced thoughts of terminating therapy even when I knew there was more work to be done.
29	0	1	2	3	4	I have questioned whether or not the reported trauma history was the real cause of my client(s) problems.
30	0	1	2	3	4	I have experienced fears that my trauma client(s) condition will have a "contagious" effect on me.
31	0	1	2	3	4	I have wished that prescribed medications would make my trauma client(s) easier to work with.
32	0	1	2	3	4	I have thought that my client(s) trauma story was not as bad as they reported it to be.
33	0	1	2	3	4	I have found "haunted" with my client(s) and their trauma history.
34	0	1	2	3	4	I have had strong emotional reactions to my trauma client(s) that lasted well beyond our meeting together.
35	0	1	2	3	4	I have felt a strong urge to solve the problems of my trauma client(s).
36	0	1	2	3	4	I have experienced a protective attitude toward my trauma client(s).
37	0	1	2	3	4	I have felt like liberator or savior in my helping role.
38	0	1	2	3	4	I have felt that working with trauma clients is really quite easy.
39	0	1	2	3	4	I have thought of my client(s) as heroic for enduring their traumatic experience.
40	0	1	2	3	4	I have done more for my trauma client(s) than is actually required by my profession.
41	0	1	2	3	4	I have been so emotionally charged from working with my trauma client(s) that it seemed as if I were the victim to.
42	0	1	2	3	4	I have found myself reliving my client(s) flashbacks, dreams or traumatic memories.
43	0	1	2	3	4	During meetings with my trauma client(s), I have found myself struggling to maintain a professional role.
44	0	1	2	3	4	During or after meeting with my trauma client(s), I have experienced headaches.
45	0	1	2	3	4	After meeting with my trauma client(s), I have experienced an inability to fall asleep or stay asleep though the nl.
46	0	1	2	3	4	I have experienced greater irritability and proneness to anger after meeting with my trauma client(s).
47	0	1	2	3	4	I have found myself using more alcohol and/or drugs after meeting with my trauma client(s).
48	0	1	2	3	4	I have experienced more stress and tension after meeting with my trauma client(s).
49	0	1	2	3	4	Meetings with trauma client(s) have been stressful.
50	0	1	2	3	4	I have experienced somatic reactions (e.g. bodily pain, throat constriction, muscle tension.) during or after session.
51	0	1	2	3	4	I have found myself growing drowsy or sleepy while listening to my trauma client(s).

	Never	Rarely	Sometimes	Often	Always	
52	0	1	2	3	4	I have experienced myself "numbing out" while listening to my trauma client(s).
53	0	1	2	3	4	I have experienced changes in my breathing pattern while listening to the trauma story of my client(s).
54	0	1	2	3	4	I have experienced nausea while listening to the trauma story of my client(s).
55	0	1	2	3	4	I have found it difficult to concentrate on my client(s) trauma story as it was being told.
56	0	1	2	3	4	I have found myself reacting as my trauma client(s) might (e.g., exaggerated startle response, on edge In crowds.)
57	0	1	2	3	4	I have found myself to be less trusting of strangers, since meeting with my trauma client(s).
58	0	1	2	3	4	I have harbored resentment of my trauma client(s) for exposing me to the pain of their suffering.
59	0	1	2	3	4	After meeting with my trauma client(s), I have found myself to be hypervigilant of what Is happening around me.
60	0	1	2	3	4	I have experienced disillusionment about the human condition due to work with trauma clients.
61	0	1	2	3	4	Due to the impact of my trauma client(s), I have found myself reappraising my own beliefs and values.
62	0	1	2	3	4	I have found myself "steering" the conversation with trauma client(s) In the direction that makes me feel least distressed.
63	0	1	2	3	4	After meeting with trauma client(s), I have difficulty getting the image of their trauma story out of my mind.
64	0	1	2	3	4	I have felt "as if" I were reliving the experiences of my trauma client(s).
65	0	1	2	3	4	After meeting with trauma clients, I experience difficulty telling others about the emotional impact of the "work" I do.
66	0	1	2	3	4	After meeting with my trauma client(s), I have experienced a loss of interest In activities that I previously enjoyed.
67	0	1	2	3	4	I have felt a need to be alone or isolated from others, after meeting with my trauma client(s).
68	0	1	2	3	4	After being exposed to trauma stories, I have experienced more concern about the safety of those I hold dear.
69	0	1	2	3	4	After meeting with trauma clients, I have experienced a sense that my life could be short or shortened prematurely.
70	0	1	2	3	4	I have experienced frustration or anger that society has not done more to prevent abuse and victimization.
71	0	1	2	3	4	I have found myself having thoughts about avenging the wrongs committed against my trauma client(s).
72	0	1	2	3	4	After meeting with my trauma client(s), I have felt overwhelmed that there is evil abuse, and victimization in the world.
73	0	1	2	3	4	I have not felt safe or trusting enough of my colleagues to be able to talk about my work and experience with trauma clients.
74	0	1	2	3	4	Due to my work with trauma clients, I have felt alienated from others who do not understand the work.
75	0	1	2	3	4	I have felt a lack of internal and/or external support in my work with trauma survivors.

	Never	Rarely	Sometimes	Often	Always	
76	0	1	2	3	4	After working with my trauma client(s). I have been preoccupied with thoughts and feelings about trauma and abuse.
77	0	1	2	3	4	Due to my work with trauma clients, I have experienced a deepened search for meaning as to why victimization occurs.
78	0	1	2	3	4	I have experienced difficulty remembering all that my trauma client(s) have told me.
79	0	1	2	3	4	Because of my work with trauma clients, I have felt a deepened sense of sadness at what some people are capable of doing.
80	0	1	2	3	4	I have found it difficult to disclose information to others about the horrific traumatic events I learn of through my work.
81	0	1	2	3	4	I have felt I cannot burden others with the traumatic events I have heard, so I keep them to myself and deal with them alone.
82	0	1	2	3	4	Since working with trauma, I have felt that I am different now from how I was before I started the work.
83	0	1	2	3	4	I have experienced feelings of grief, mourning, and sadness during or after meeting with my trauma client(s).
84	0	1	2	3	4	In my work with trauma clients, I have experienced "being out of touch" with my own emotions or feelings.
85	0	1	2	3	4	I have experienced a loss of sensuality and emotional sensitivity due to my immersion in trauma work.
86	0	1	2	3	4	The impact of the trauma work has caused me to feel "as if" I were living in a bad dream with surreal features.
87	0	1	2	3	4	In my professional work with trauma, I have experienced vicarious traumatization.
88	0	1	2	3	4	I have found that my trauma clients heal very quickly.
89	0	1	2	3	4	I am touched by my trauma clients and their stories.
90	0	1	2	3	4	I have been reluctant to speak honestly to colleagues/supervisors for fear of being viewed as novice: Inept or wrong.
91	0	1	2	3	4	I have felt abandoned by my supervisors or colleagues in Issues with my trauma clients.
92	0	1	2	3	4	I have felt threatened or unsafe due to the behavior(s) of my trauma client(s).
93	0	1	2	3	4	I have experienced fear of my trauma client(s).
94	0	1	2	3	4	I have fantasized that I would feel safer if indeed my client(s) went through with through with their threaten suicide or were dead.
95	0	1	2	3	4	I have experienced an adrenaline rush or high while working with trauma clients.
96	0	1	2	3	4	I have experienced heightened sense of meaning or reason for being when I do trauma work.
97	0	1	2	3	4	I believe that PTSD Is being over used as a diagnosis for other types of problems.
98	0	1	2	3	4	I have felt that many clients over-react to their trauma, utilizing histrionic reactions to perceived Injury.
99	0	1	2	3	4	I believe that many clients malinger or fake their PTSD or trauma symptoms.
100	0	1	2	3	4	Due to the nature of my work with trauma clients, I secretly wish I were doing something else with my career.

Comments and reactions related to your experience completing the Clinicians' Trauma Reaction Survey (CTRS) are appreciated in the space below. Once again, our thanks to you!

_____

_____

_____

_____

_____

Instructions

Some professionals report somatic changes or occurrences related to their work with trauma survivors. Please read the following and circle the number that best applies to your experience.

1. Your gender:
   (a) FEMALE
   (b) MALE

2. Your present age:
   (a) 25 or less
   (b) 26–35
   (c) 36–45
   (d) 46–55
   (e) 56–65
   (f) 66 or greater

3. Your ethnic/cultural heritage:
   (a) Asian
   (b) Black/African American
   (c) Hispanic
   (d) Native American/Alaskan Native
   (e) White/European American
   (f) Other (please specify) _____

4. Your belief or faith category:
   (a) Spiritual (non-secular, higher power)
   (b) Christian (Catholic Protestant)
   (c) Judaism
   (d) Eastern Religion; (Buddhist Hindu)
   (e) Atheist (no spiritual or religious belief)
   (f) Other (please specify) _____

5. Highest level of education (circle highest level achieved):
   (a) undergraduate degree
   (b) masters degree
   (c) doctoral degree
   (d) professional medical degree

   (e) other (please specify) _____

6. License/Credentials (circle all that apply):
   (a) MSW
   (b) ISW
   (c) ICSW
   (d) DSW
   (e) LPO
   (f) LPCC/LMHC
   (g) Ph.D
   (h) Psy.D
   (i) M.D
   (j) D.O.
   (k) RNLPN/NP
   (l) MDIV
   (m) DDJV
   (n) JD/LLB
   (o) Other (specify)_____

7. Your number of years experience in a helping profession (Include internship/residency):
   (a) 1–5 years
   (b) 8–10 years
   (c) 11–15 years
   (d) 16–20 years
   (e) 21 years or more

8. Note your years of experience working with trauma clients:
   (a) 1–5 years
   (b) 6–10 years
   (c) 11–15 years
   (d) 16–20 years
   (e) 21 years or more

9. Note the average percentage per year of trauma related clients you treat or assess:
   (a) 0%/year
   (b) 1–10%/year
   (c) 11–25%/year
   (d) 28–50%/year
   (e) 51–75%/year
   (f) 76–100%/year

10. Note your hours per week of work with trauma clients:
    (a) 0–5 hours/week
    (b) 6–10 hours/week
    (c) 11–20 hours/week
    (d) 21–30 hours/week
    (e) 31–40 hours/week
    (f) 41 or more hours

11. Note the hours per month of peer counseling/supervision you participate in:
    (a) 0 hours per month
    (b) 1–2 hours per month
    (c) 3–5 hours per month
    (d) 6–10 hours per month
    (e) 11 or more hours per month

12. Note your training in treatment of Post Traumatic Stress Disorder (circle all that apply):
    (a) academic classes
    (b) internship/residency
    (c) seminars/conferences
    (d) other (please specify)_____
    (e) no training

13. Who do you talk with about your feelings and/or the nature of your work with trauma clients and how much do you share? (Answer I & II)

    I. PEOPLE YOU SHARE WITH
        (circle all that apply)
    (a) Supervisor ....(0) none
    (b) Colleague........................(0) none
    (c) Spouse/Significant
        Other ....(0) none
    (d) Minister, Priest,
        Rabbi, etc. ....(0) none
    (e) Family member ....(0) none
    (f) Friend.............................(0) none
    (g) Other (specify)_____
    (h) I do not share with anyone, I keep the impact of my work to myself.

II. DEGREE TO WHICH YOU SHARE
     (circle all that apply)
     (1) Small   (2) Moderate   (3) Great
     (1) Small   (2) Moderate   (3) Great
     (1) Small   (2) Moderate   (3) Great
     (1) Small   (2) Moderate   (3) Great
     (1) Small   (2) Moderate   (3) Great
     (1) Small   (2) Moderate   (3) Great
     (1) Small   (2) Moderate   (3) Great

14. Please note the trauma population(s) you work with (circle all that apply):
    (1) War Veteran
    (2) Civilian Survivor of War
    (3) Holocaust Survivor
    (4) Family of Holocaust Survivor
    (5) Refugee
    (6) Political Tyranny, Torture Victims
    (7) Sexual Assault—adult
    (8) Childhood Sexual Abuse
    (9) Physical Abuse—child/adult
    (10) Battered Spouse/Significant Other
    (11) Emotional Abuse—child/adult
    (12) Attempted Suicide
    (13) Medical Trauma (surgery, illness)
    (14) Severe personal injury
    (15) Occupational Trauma (medic, police …)
    (16) Transport Disaster (car, plane, train, bus)
    (17) Natural Disaster
    (18) Technological Disaster
    (19) Stalking, Abduction, Highjack, Hostage
    (20) Traumatic Separation (from parent, family)
    (21) Victim of Violent Crime (robbery, mugging)
    (22) Witness of Violence (crime, injury, suicide)
    (23) Sexual or Gender identity/ Orientation
    (24) Other (please specify) _____

15. Please note the trauma population(s) you would refer to other professionals (circle all that apply):
    (1) War Veteran
    (2) Civilian Survivor of War
    (3) Holocaust Survivor
    (4) Family of Holocaust Survivor
    (5) Refugee
    (6) Political Tyranny, Torture Victims

(7) Sexual Assault adult
(8) Childhood Sexual Abuse
(9) Physical Abuse—child/adult
(10) Battered Spouse/Significant Other
(11) Emotional Abuse—child/adult
(12) Attempted Suicide
(13) Medical Trauma (Surgery, illness)
(14) Severe personal injury
(15) Occupational Trauma (medic, polices ...)
(16) Transport Disaster (car, plane, train, bus)
(17) Natural Disaster
(18) Technological Disaster
(19) Stalking Abduction Highjack, Hostage
(20) Traumatic separation (from parent family)
(21) Victim of Violent Crime (robbery, smuggling)
(22) Witness of Violence (crime, injury, suicide)
(23) Sexual or Gender Identity/ Orientation
(24) Other (please specify) _____

16. Do you have a personal trauma history?
    (a) No   (b) Yes   (if yes, circle from the list below)
    (1) War Veteran
    (2) Civilian Survivor of War
    (3) Holocaust Survivor
    (4) Family of Holocaust Survivor
    (5) Refugee
    (6) Political Tyranny Torture Victims
    (7) Sexual Assault adult
    (8) Childhood Sexual Abuse
    (9) Physical Abuser child/adult
    (10) Battered Spouse/Significant Other
    (11) Emotional Abuse-child/adult
    (12) Attempted Suicide
    (13) Medical Trauma (Surgery, illness)
    (14) Severe personal injury
    (15) Occupational Trauma (medic, police ...)
    (16) Transport Disaster (car, plane, train, bus)
    (17) Natural Disaster

(18) Technological Disaster
(19) Stalking Abduction High Jack, Hostage
(20) Traumatic separation (from parent family)
(21) Victim of Violent Crime (robbery, smuggling)
(22) Witness of Violence (crime, injury, suicide)
(23) Sexual or Gender Identity/ Orientation
(24) Other (please specify) _____

17. Please note the types of trauma related behavior you would prefer to refer to other professionals (circle all that apply):
    (1) Self Mutilation (cutting, burning)
    (2) Attempted Suicide
    (3) Dissociative Episodes
    (4) Excessive Drug/Alcohol Abuse
    (5) Flashbacks
    (6) Night Terrors
    (7) Eating Disorders (bulimia, anorexia)
    (8) Violent Crime (history/police record)
    (9) Perpetrator—Adult (history/police record)
    (10) Perpetrator—Child (history/police record)
    (11) Stalking Behavior (history/police record)
    (12) Possession of Weapons
    (13) Borderline Characteristics
    (14) Antisocial Behavior
    (15) Menacing Violent, Rageful
    (16) Disruptive/Oppositional Behavior
    (17) Ritualistic Abusive Behavior
    (18) Thrill Seeking Behavior
    (19) Major Depressive Behavior
    (20) Sexually Seductive Behavior
    (21) Extreme Isolation & Detachment
    (22) Disfunctional Family Behavior
    (23) Other (please specify) _____

18. On a scale of 0 (none) to 4 (extremely) to what degree is your spiritual or religious belief system a support to you in this work? (circle one) (0) (1) (2) (3) (4)

Index